How to Cut It in the Media

A PR Manual for Aesthetic Plastic Surgeons
& Professionals in Cosmetic Medicine

Tingy Simoes
Owner and MD of Marketing
and PR agency, Wavelength
Marketing Communications,
London, UK

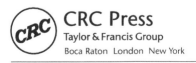

CRC Press
Taylor & Francis Group
Boca Raton London New York

CRC Press is an imprint of the
Taylor & Francis Group, an **informa** business

CRC Press
Taylor & Francis Group
6000 Broken Sound Parkway NW, Suite 300
Boca Raton, FL 33487-2742

© 2013 by Taylor & Francis Group, LLC
CRC Press is an imprint of Taylor & Francis Group, an Informa business

No claim to original U.S. Government works

Printed on acid-free paper
Version Date: 20130731

International Standard Book Number-13: 978-1-84214-549-4 (Paperback)

This book contains information obtained from authentic and highly regarded sources. While all reasonable efforts have been made to publish reliable data and information, neither the author[s] nor the publisher can accept any legal responsibility or liability for any errors or omissions that may be made. The publishers wish to make clear that any views or opinions expressed in this book by individual editors, authors or contributors are personal to them and do not necessarily reflect the views/opinions of the publishers. The information or guidance contained in this book is intended for use by medical, scientific or health-care professionals and is provided strictly as a supplement to the medical or other professional's own judgement, their knowledge of the patient's medical history, relevant manufacturer's instructions and the appropriate best practice guidelines. Because of the rapid advances in medical science, any information or advice on dosages, procedures or diagnoses should be independently verified. The reader is strongly urged to consult the drug companies' printed instructions, and their websites, before administering any of the drugs recommended in this book. This book does not indicate whether a particular treatment is appropriate or suitable for a particular individual. Ultimately it is the sole responsibility of the medical professional to make his or her own professional judgements, so as to advise and treat patients appropriately. The authors and publishers have also attempted to trace the copyright holders of all material reproduced in this publication and apologize to copyright holders if permission to publish in this form has not been obtained. If any copyright material has not been acknowledged please write and let us know so we may rectify in any future reprint.

Visit the Taylor & Francis Web site at
http://www.taylorandfrancis.com

and the CRC Press Web site at
http://www.crcpress.com

Contents

About the Author		iv
Acknowledgements and Publisher's Note		vi
1.	Introduction	1
2.	Why talk to the press?	7
3.	What do we mean by public relations?	12
4.	Reactive PR	18
5.	Proactive PR	27
6.	What is newsworthy?	31
7.	Knowing your audience (or Don't try and get down wit' da kidz)	50
8.	Tools of the trade	60
9.	Pitching to journalists	73
10.	Interview techniques	85
11.	Social media	104
12.	Conclusions	109
Index		117

About the Author

Tingy Simoes is owner and MD of Marketing and PR agency Wavelength Marketing Communications and has extensive experience from the world of PR for medical professionals in both the UK and the USA.

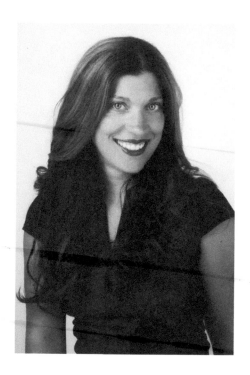

If you ask my 8 year old what mummy does for a living, he'll say "she puts doctors on television," and I suppose, rather crudely, that is what Public Relations entails—only I also help them get into magazines, newspapers and radio. If further queried, he might explain (probably giggling) that a lot of these doctors "make people's bums smaller" …

Tingy's career spans across three continents and over fifteen years of Marketing Communications. A native Venezuelan, she began work in New York City as Director of Marketing for a financial PR consultancy and later moved into a healthcare-focused agency where she was quickly promoted up the ranks. During this time she worked with clients varying from heart monitors and diabetes products to medical credentialing and cosmetic surgery.

Headhunted to run the internal branding and graphic design unit at Goldman Sachs International, Tingy moved to London but eventually decided to launch her own consultancy, Wavelength Marketing Communications. Now in its 10th year, Wavelength has helped establish a number of high-profile organisations as the most respected voices in healthcare, as well as managed high-pressure projects such as steering the British Association of Aesthetic Plastic Surgeons Press Office through the PIP implants crisis and announcing to the world's media the groundbreaking separation of craniopagus twins by children's charity Facing the World.

The success of Wavelength was swiftly followed by the introduction of a sister PR agency also focused on healthcare, Cacique Public Relations, in 2006. Cacique, pronounced *ka'seek* meaning 'leader of the tribe' also grew exponentially, representing a wide range of private enterprises both in the UK and abroad – from hospitals and clinics to high-tech products and medical devices such as lasers, skincare brands and even implants. Both agencies regularly achieve hundreds of placements in the UK and international media on a regular basis, from the BBC and Al Jazeera, to Reuters, the Wall Street Journal and the New York Times as well as top women's glossies.

An avid public speaker, Tingy has addressed audiences at business networking events and seminars, major healthcare conferences and even lectured on entrepreneurship and marketing for a career development programme for Ph.D students at Cambridge University.

Tingy regularly writes articles for a number of healthcare trade magazines, and holds a degree in Business Administration and Marketing from the New School University in New York City.

Acknowledgements

So this is the bit where I list a bunch of names that mean little to anyone else but a lot to me ...

I owe a huge debt of thanks to my lovely colleagues Kate Chaundy, Steve Bustin and my deranged new assistant Nikki Milovanovic—without them holding the fort I would never have been able to finish this project. Here's also a shout-out to the many fantastic journalists I've worked with over the years such as Barney Calman, Jo MacFarlane, Fiona Macrae, Matt Barbour, Leah Hardy, Alice Smellie, Alice Hart-Davis, Jeremy Laurance, Chris Smyth, Caroline Crowe, Katherine Jarman, Lorna Jackson, Chris Choi, Melanie Abbot, Madeleine Lown and everyone at *Newsbeat* as well as the delightful and ever-wise Rebecca Smith. There are simply too many names to mention here, but know that having a laugh with you guys keeps me going! Kind thanks also are due to Vicky Eldridge from *Cosmetic News* and Robin Stride at *Independent Practitioner Today* for allowing me to re-use articles written for them. Special mention must go to my very dear friend and groundbreaking cosmetic surgery reporter (HRH) Joan Kron.

A massive thank you to Robert Peden at Informa who believed in my modest proposal; to all my clients including Leonor Stepjic at RAFT (been a long time coming!); and in particular to the BAAPS for giving me a chance when I first launched the good ship Wavelength over a decade ago—Norman, Adam, Douglas, Nigel, Fazel and Rajiv, it's been a privilege serving alongside you gentlemen, and long may our relationship continue.

By far the biggest thanks of all go to my family, who are driven utterly mad by my relentless 24/7 job yet with loving patience manage to keep me just on the threshold of sane.

PUBLISHER'S NOTE

The material in the Introduction was originally published as 'Botox Babylon' in *Cosmetic News* magazine, and is reprinted with kind permission.

Much of the material in the section 'Communicating in the PIP crisis ...' in Chapter 12 was originally published as 'Lessons extracted from the PIP crisis' in *Independent Practitioner Today*, and is reprinted with kind permission.

1 Introduction

It's difficult to encompass just how much the industry and people's expectations surrounding cosmetic surgery and aesthetic treatments have changed in the last ten years. But I'm sure that most practitioners, publicists (and the public itself) would agree that there's clearly been an increase in hysterical reporting in the consumer press, with journalists on a never-ending quest for what's new, sexy, lurid and bizarre.

Some people in our industry may recognise my name, possibly because it's rather odd, but also because they know me as the publicist for organisations such as the British Association of Aesthetic Plastic Surgeons and the British Academy of Cosmetic Dentistry, although I have worked on both sides of the Atlantic. Over the last decade my team and I have also helped launch a wide range of now-recognisable brands including lasers, skincare products, medical devices and even implants.

In my role as Press Officer I have had to field my share of ludicrous press enquiries. One memorable example was a journalist undergoing breast reduction for a documentary; she wanted to know if she could "cremate the removed tissue into a diamond", or could I suggest something 'wacky' to do with it. I contemplated a list including 'Stir fry' and 'Knit into a hat' but forced myself to explain it's incinerated as a biohazard.

I've been asked whether a buxom glamour model's implants can melt during a jungle-based reality TV show, and what would happen if a mosquito bit her breast (I actually don't know—would the mosquito die …?). I recently took a call from a weight loss-related documentary, where the producer asked "if I could bike them over some fat", so the contestants could gain perspective on how much they'd lost throughout the series. Naturally the answer was an emphatic 'no' (do they think I keep a minibar in the office for this kind of thing?).

All of this clearly demonstrates that (i) I have a strange job and (ii) there continues to be an intense fascination in the world of cosmetic surgery which presents tremendous opportunities for key players who want to promote themselves to the media.

These last ten turbulent years have seen scandalised headlines on subjects ranging from trout pouts and pillow faces, to 'exploding' breast implants, moobs and deadly buttock injections. I believe that my experiences have taught me what works for the press, and what doesn't, which allows me to offer you some useful dos and don'ts for your own public relations (PR) campaigns.

As the Noughties introduced us to Google, text messaging and Ugg boots, journalists in the mainstream media seemed grateful for pretty much any titbit (pardon the pun) from the hitherto 'secret' and privileged world of facelifts, liposuction and Botox. These procedures are still perceived as the prerogative of only the rich and famous, and publicity could be garnered with somewhat relative ease. Offering general comment on the advent of makeover shows, for example, or a warning against going abroad for cheap surgery deals were (and still are) legitimate ways to secure press interest, especially if there's anything controversial in the views being expressed, and if they can 'piggyback' on something topical that's already in the news.

I have found three approaches that will, almost always, 'hook' journalists' interest. The first is rather obvious and probably one of the easiest sells: 'new' procedures, techniques or technology. Most magazines and newspapers are continually on the lookout for what's new and, unfortunately for the reputation of the industry as a whole, a lot of the time they don't seem to care whether it actually works or not. I've managed some very successful stories surrounding new applications of traditional techniques, such as for turkey necks, back rolls and muffin-tops (sometimes I think I could swap press releases with a bakery!), but I've also seen some distasteful press releases—not my own, I hasten to add—crash and burn. 'Speedo Sag' just sounds gross, and quite frankly to insinuate that women are getting more Botox during the Super Bowl/World Cup because 'they're not allowed at home' during the games is plain misogynistic.

Announcing a new tweak on an existing treatment and giving it a groovy new name, isn't, in itself, wrong (these aren't just ANY veneers …). When done well (e.g. the technique was published in a medical journal; it taps into a current trend; you have a willing case study with strong before-and-after photography), it's probably the closest you'll ever come to actually guaranteeing coverage.

However, for this to work the procedure should *actually be new*, and, most importantly, proven to work. From the Miami Thong Lift to the Snap-On Celebrity Smile there must, in reality, be something different and effective as well as 'new'. This is why so many supposed procedures that are meant to be 'the latest craze from Hollywood' come and go, never to be heard of again. To this day I'm still being hounded by journalists trying to locate the apparent hordes of women undergoing dimpleplasty to look like pop star Cheryl Cole, or shoulder lipo (maybe for a story titled *Tormented by My Fat Clavicles*).

The second area extremely likely to garner exposure includes statistics, research studies and trends. There is some leeway here to allow you to get creative and we will explore them in detail—though unfortunately the pressure PR agencies are under to deliver coverage has resulted in some real howlers. Most respectable outlets will query a claim of '300% rise', because they suspect it means three patients. I've lost count of the amount of times that journalists will call me to check whether it's really true that there's been a 40% rise in patients having 'Blackberry Botox' or 'Revenge Surgery'. You must be willing and able to prove and defend statistics you put out to the media.

Trends and warnings work well. If, say, your practice is seeing more temporomandibular disorder patients than usual, it is certainly worth positing a theory that people may be grinding more due to worries in the recession, and drafting a genuine warning on how to prevent the problem.

Finally, there's human interest … the absolute ideal. But WHY, many of my clients demand, this obsession with case studies? Can't the journalists just *take my word for it?* In a word: no. I'm sure I don't have to tell you how competitive it's become out there. Everyone is offering aesthetic treatments (whether they're appropriately trained and qualified is a whole other kettle of fillers) and it's becoming very difficult to differentiate. Basically, if you say you're good, you'll need to prove it. Journalists want patient stories that illustrate the impact of your care and talents—the more dramatic the story, the better. It's no use ranting at your poor publicists because they can't get a lip augmentation case study placed on the cover of *Cosmopolitan!*

While I'm on the theme of case studies, allow me the indulgence of a small rant about photography. Why is it that so many clinics and practitioners fail to take good pictures of their patients? I have received so many photos where I literally cannot tell which is the 'before' and which is the 'after'. I know of a clinic that still takes only Polaroids! Photos are what sell the story. They must be high resolution, and represent 'like to like'. If the patient is smiling in the 'before', he/she should be smiling in the 'after'. A laser lipo story, where the 'before' photo shows the patient leaning forward but standing and sucking in the tummy in the 'after' photo will not make it into the paper unless the case study can come up with some candid (maybe on holiday in a swimsuit) shots where the difference is not only discernible but also drastic. Also, a slight reality check: your 65-year-old male patient will never make it into *GQ*.

This brings me to one last, but essential, aspect that must be considered by those of you looking to explore, launch, continue or revisit a PR campaign whether in-house or with an agency: ensure you have an understanding of the outlets you're trying to target, their age groups and their audience demographics. So many times

I have been told by clients (whilst wrinkling their delicate noses) that their patients 'simply do not read the tabloids'. Instead, they feel it would be best to educate the readers of the *Financial Times* about preventing wrinkles and tooth decay. Might I suggest that for the readers of those august publications that horse has already bolted?

So what, in the media's view, makes the perfect story? One that combines all the above, of course! A catchy headline, perhaps a celebrity or celebrity 'hooks', some strong statistics, a case study with a legitimately new procedure and a strong emotional back-story … or at least, one with some of those elements. Perhaps, if cosmetic surgery and aesthetic treatment providers can all increase the quality and the content of their communications, we might be able to better educate and reach the media and thereby the public.

I sure would miss those crazy media enquiries though.

WHY THIS BOOK?

With the advent of 24-hour news cycles, the requirement for expert comment in the media has exploded. Medical spokespeople are regularly approached to demystify new technology and advances, or give their learned opinion regarding the latest developments. Specifically in cosmetic surgery and medicine, relatively lax regulation has led to a proliferation of unscrupulous behaviour, aggressive marketing and a rise in horror stories about people going to backstreet clinics for everything from Botox to buttock enhancement—creating an urgent, ever-increasing need for reputable spokespeople to provide reliable guidance and advice to the public.

This book will cover both 'Reactive' media relations, that is, when the press needs (usually urgently) comment from a clinician or professional in the aesthetic arena and 'Proactive' media relations, that is, when physicians themselves voluntarily seek to liaise with the media to either highlight an issue of public interest, or raise their own personal profiles.

This handy how-to guide will outline why it's important to be prepared for either approach, and provides potential spokespeople with comprehensive advice on the best way to communicate with journalists, as well as suggestions on how to avoid the most common pitfalls. I will also be outlining the pros and cons of 'sticking one's head above the parapet' and offer tips on dealing with a wide variety of outlets: trade versus consumer press, national versus regional, encompassing print, radio, television and the latest in social media. There is guidance on interviews and how to deal with difficult, intrusive or even accusatory questions.

As in any area of marketing, publicity can also catastrophically fail, and I will highlight examples where industry players—whether practitioners, clinics or even governmental organisations—drop the ball in so spectacular a fashion that business schools of the future will probably use them as case studies in their 'PR blunders' module.

2 Why talk to the press?

At their most basic, aesthetic professionals (whether clinicians such as doctors, surgeons, dermatologists, nurses, dentists or clinic and hospital owners/managers) can be divided into two types: (i) those who actively seek to interact with the media—whether to advance their own profiles or generate business—and (ii) those that feel the limelight is thrust upon them in spite of their wishes or inclination. They see the press as a 'necessary evil' and mistrust journalists. Either way, to ignore the power of the press in today's media-led society is foolhardy. This handbook will provide the tools and insider knowledge to take ownership of your PR endeavours, in whichever of those camps you consider yourself to be.

Under what circumstances would a journalist ever need or want to speak with you? The answer is EVERY time they write or report anything having to do with aesthetic treatments or news in the sector, they will need comment from 'an expert'. I've lost count of the amount of times I have been asked by industry players: "What is *that* clown doing on TV?" The reality is that whether you agree or not that the person they end up using actually qualifies as an expert, it doesn't change that ultimately the media needs someone—anyone—to quote and give their story validity. And for better or for worse, the selection of expert mainly comes down to one thing: PR. Either you enjoy the relationship yourself with a journalist, or have a publicist with the right connections ... or you don't!

> *You may choose not to proactively engage with the press, but to ignore the power of the media is more than disingenuous, it's outright stupid.*

On the other hand, there are dumb reasons to hire a PR agency and one of them is simply wanting to 'be on television'. I've met experts throughout my career who feel that they entirely missed their calling and actually they just want to appear on TV chat shows. They don't technically have a unique viewpoint, or any specific news to impart, but feel they themselves are a gift of greatness to be unleashed upon an unsuspecting world. This has a short lifespan as a PR strategy. We might be able to get you on a couple of programmes here and there, but there must be substance behind the gloss and actual value to provide to the media. If you want your life to be more *Entourage* than *Scrubs*, consider getting an agent.

Another no-good reason—doomed to fail, in fact—to engage a PR agency is because you actually want to spend less time on marketing. A PR agency will need you to provide material to take to the press and we require your involvement and commitment. To every client I say: "I'm only as good as what you give me." Having a PR agency will not reduce your hours, if anything quite the opposite, but it will multiply your rewards in terms of recognition.

WHAT THEY NEED FROM YOU

So why does the media need you? Because, make no mistake, **they need you**. They require:

- Information
- Explanation
- Illumination
- Expertise and knowledge
- Opinion

The press just wants a good story! The sooner every medical spokesperson arrives at the understanding that a journalist's job is simply to produce one, the easier it will be to deal with the media on a regular basis. It is the underlying reasoning and objective to everything they do. Know that journalists are NOT there to inform, rally, reassure, educate or inspire for the greater good. They are not there to make the human race better people, promote safety or encourage commonsense decision-making: their mission is to sell newspapers and magazines, and get their viewer and listener figures up. This is their job. And anyone who helps them to look good in front of their boss will earn their gratitude and a fruitful, long-term relationship.

> *Make it snappy! If you can make sensible advice and viewpoints sound interesting or appealing, you're halfway there.*

CELEBRITY DOCTORS

With advances in the sector and new aesthetic treatments being touted everyday as the 'latest craze from Hollywood', the urgent need for expert view has risen exponentially. As the new century dawned, a new phenomenon was also making its way into our collective consciousness: the meteoric rise of the celebrity doctor. Of the hundreds of physicians I have worked with over the years my team and I always knew who were the media stars (or 'media sluts', as some of their colleagues more rudely put it) who were willing to do interviews anytime, no matter how obscure the outlet.

Suddenly the public knew the names of doctors and knew them well—from dramatic makeover shows to reality 'fly in the wall' documentaries—the fact that certain medical luminaries had chosen to descend from the perceived Olympian heights of their consulting rooms and walk/Twitter among the common folk was regarded by the media as nothing short of manna from heaven. Suddenly you could call them by their first names, you knew what they ate for breakfast and they also shared their fitness tips. The most successful ones not only publish books but they're also on TV, Facebook and Twitter. Clearly it doesn't translate that they're necessarily better at what they do than any of their colleagues, but just that they know how to harness the power of media in their favour. In particular, the cosmetic surgery sector, having been seen until relatively recently as the preserve of the rich and famous and somewhat shrouded in an aura of mystery, became one of the areas most sensationalised in the press. A succession of makeover shows exploded onto our screens, showing us what transformations could be achieved. We read in magazines who did so-and-so's facelift, so-and-so's boobs. In some circles, surgery has started to be seen as a badge of honour and some patients *want* acquaintances to ask "who did your nose?"

Doctors, surgeons and professionals in aesthetic health care eventually woke to this dawning reality—some more quickly than others—and jumped into frenzied marketing and publicity activity with gusto but rather mixed results. The 'Wild West' analogy is used quite often to describe the sector, as providers of aesthetic treatments can seem untroubled by much in the way of statutory limitations on what they can and can't do. The reality is that, whether provided by board certified, appropriately trained and qualified practitioners or not, the idea of cosmetic surgery has become firmly entrenched in today's popular culture. There is even a sense of entitlement among the public, with many feeling they 'deserve' a little pick-me-up in the form of wrinkle-relaxing injections or a neck lift in the same way they view having a haircut. One could posit the theory that the ubiquity of cosmetic surgery advertising and marketing has contributed to its trivialisation in the eyes of the public, leading to their own dangerous undoing in many cases.

It is in this environment that it's more important than ever that reputable clinicians make themselves heard. Sometimes even those dead set against the idea of interacting with the press ('whoring' themselves out) in any way may still be forced to give statements to the media if they're involved in a high-profile case, or they're— God forbid—'doorstepped'. We will be looking at the difference between 'reactive' and 'proactive' PR in an upcoming chapter.

The reasons for engaging with the press should be clear. Below-the-line marketing (known this way historically because it is not a direct cost like buying an advert, which is considered 'Above the Line') such as Public Relations is done mainly to foster awareness and generate goodwill from the press, thereby gaining recognition and valuable mind 'real estate' among their audiences. Whether ultimately it's because you want to drive patients to your private practice/clinic, or you want to warn or educate the public about certain trends or dangers, the result of engaging with them is that the media get to know you. The more you make yourself available, the more they'll call upon you.

It's a well-known marketing adage that, if you don't seek to secure a position yourself, your competitors and customers will do it for you. Start thinking of PR like going to the gym: paying your membership alone isn't going to get you any benefits! You need to invest more than money; think creatively, engage and commit to the cause. You know that, if you do, you could be looking pretty hot just a few months from now …

3 What do we mean by public relations?

"HI, I'M GREAT IN BED."

There are several versions of this anecdote, but it does illustrate quite well how PR fits into the marketing mix (for the purposes of this example, you are a heterosexual male):

- You see an attractive woman at a party. You go up to her and say "Hi, I'm great in bed!" This is Direct Marketing.
- You see an attractive woman at a party. You pay someone to walk up to her, point at you and say "My friend is great in bed." This is Advertising.
- You see an attractive woman at a party. You befriend people she trusts, take them out to dinner and convince them to talk to her about how great you are in bed. This is Public Relations.
- You're at a party and an attractive woman comes to you and says "I hear you're great in bed." This is the power of Branding.

Real branding is successfully secured when your name has become synonymous with something in the public's perception; whether it's cutting edge procedures, celebrity connections or having a facelift technique named after you. It can only be achieved through proactive marketing and this includes, invariably, PR efforts.

There are rules and guidelines—varying in strictness and specificity—as to how a medical professional can approach prospects, although like any code these can be and are occasionally flouted. There is no point in reviewing unethical ways of contacting possible patients—in this book, we will be sticking with securing media endorsement.

I began my career in health care PR during the dot-com boom, when budgets were plentiful, and a new generation of companies with brightly coloured walls and skateboarding CEOs knew to invest in making as much noise as possible. Appearing in the *New York Times* or *Marie Claire* magazine was—and continues to be—of paramount importance. But even as the bountiful 90s gave way to the more restrained Noughties, one reality remained: the comparative cost of retaining a PR agency versus booking expensive adverts in magazines and newspapers is still a no-brainer. How else could you achieve hundreds of articles with just one press release? Advertising simply cannot measure up to the reach of Public Relations. During the height of the PIP implant crisis in the U.K. (December 11–January 12), the British Association of Aesthetic Plastic Surgeons issued roughly 10 press releases which resulted in over 1500 media clippings, which if purchased as advertising, which would have cost a cool £5 million (nearly $8 million). There is simply no contest.

But in addition to the straightforward cost differences, there is the intangible value of the public's inherent trust upon the media (for better or worse). I may not believe it when a hospital tells me they are the best—I mean, of course they would say that—but I might believe *Hello!* Magazine or the *New York Times* when they do their 'top 10 cosmetic providers' list. People do not doubt that the journalists have done the research for them. Whether this is the case or not (and in many cases, sadly, it's not), the truth remains that the public believe in the guidance and recommendations of their favourite columnist or TV presenter. They value celebrity endorsement: "if that's the eye cream that Jennifer Aniston uses, well it sure as heck is going to be the one I'll be buying ..."

A few years ago a well-known chain of supermarkets decided to compile a 'Best Cosmetic Doctors' list for their popular in-house monthly magazine, generally filled with recipes and money-off coupons, sold at the tills. PR agencies around the country (including our own) went into overdrive, contacting every free-lancer involved and all the editors, sending profiles of our clients and before-and-after photography of their case studies, offering interviews and visits to the clinics. Ironically, some of our clients were fairly blasé about our efforts towards this oh-so-democratic outlet—in particular, those who generally aim for publicity in high society glossies and who believe their patients 'don't read the tabloids'. Three or four years later, they still say to us in astonished accents: "I can't believe the amount of business I got from being included in that magazine. I'm still getting patients who refer to it." Your position on Google is inarguably paramount these days. But the most effective form of marketing will combine both online and offline strategies.

> *Remember: magazines live forever, in beauty salons and doctors' offices ...!*

The 2006 Mintel market research report into cosmetic surgery stated:
"Public Relations is by far the most effective form of advertising that a clinic or hospital can undertake. Effective PR can work wonders in terms of providing consumers with information on the latest developments in the industry."

THE MARKETING MIX

Or AIDA is not just an opera

Your overall image is a composite of a whole host of Marketing Elements, some of which you may or may not make use of including branding, advertising, personal selling, special offers and promotions, packaging, sponsorships, merchandising, exhibitions/trade shows, Public Relations and word of mouth. In this book, we will be solely focused on PR, but keep in mind that your activity in this area should remain in line with all other promotional efforts that you engage in, or your brand (I hear you're great in bed) will appear disjointed.

> *Note: You cannot control word of mouth—you may seek to incentivise it with vouchers or discounts for 'refer-a-friend', but ultimately you cannot actually control what people say about you. This includes journalists!*

Particularly, the difference between Advertising and PR is the biggest area of confusion among newbies first dipping their toes into formal, proactive Marketing endeavours. They want an article in a newspaper that mentions them, and only them. They want their logo included. They want it to take up exactly one-half of a page. "Have them print a profile about me, my charity work and include photos of me with my diving/bowling/fishing trophies." Let's be clear: that is not editorial, it would be classified as straightforward advertising. In a product's (or indeed, any organisation's) life cycle, there are various channels to market which are appropriate at different stages.

At the very start, when budgets are tight, most businesses tend to rely on personal contacts, basic listings, word of mouth and referrals. But as they grow, they can explore other options such as promotions (e.g., discounts and special offers), PR and eventually leading to the most expensive approach, advertising.

In marketing, there is a well-known decision-making framework known as AIDA: Awareness, Interest, Desire and Action (the last two also known as 'Conviction' and 'Purchase'), and different marketing approaches can appeal to each of these stages of consumer consciousness in different ways. For example, advertising is the farthest reaching—nothing can beat taking out a whole page ad in a popular magazine or booking a prime-time TV commercial: it will secure more eyeballing than a mention in an article or programme (hence advertising ranks very high in fostering 'Awareness').

If your budget allows for a Super Bowl commercial, then by all means take advantage of this opportunity. However for the majority of us, the costs would be prohibitive. In addition the public are savvy, they know it's paid for, so an ad will always carry less credibility because it's technically not vetted or endorsed in any way by the magazine or shows in which it appears. If the health editor, however, mentions your product or service, it instantly carries much more weight because they are someone the readers trust. Thus, PR ranks higher in the 'Interest' and 'Desire' areas. Personal selling is the most effective at spurring a decision (i.e., 'purchase') which is why conversion rates will be influenced by how personable you are—but doctors can hardly approach people in the street and try to convince them to have a consultation if they've expressed no interest to begin with. It's a legal and ethical minefield, and should rightly be off the table for consideration.

Marketing doesn't function in a vacuum. All points of contact with patients, from ambiance in the waiting room to artwork on the walls, to packaging of any proprietary products (own skincare lines, etc.) are an opportunity to foster AIDA.

ADVERTISING	VS	EDITORIAL (PR)
You pay for the mention		The coverage is free
Full control over copy		You don't control what's written
Less credibility		More trust from the public
Date it appears is established by you		You may not necessarily know when it comes out
Only expert/clinic included is yours		Other experts may be quoted
You can include photos, logos		Will rarely, if ever, include logos
Final 'proof' is provided before print		You won't know how it looks or its context
Is not affected by external events		Space depends on other news

Some print outlets will try to sell you advertorials, a combination of both: it's the magazine or newspaper's compromise in terms of running your ad, and also writing a bit about you. In some cases, it's the only way you'll get into the publication, but this only tends to happen with certain small or local outlets. It's usually quite clear when you read an article whether it was paid for (personally, when I'm flicking through a magazine and realise it says 'PROMOTION' at the top, my eyes tend to glaze over).

As a general rule, advertising and editorial are entirely separate departments, and there's much stigma attached to being viewed as compromising journalistic 'integrity'. It would be very unusual for a national newspaper or high-end, glossy magazine to demand advertising in exchange for editorial unless it's, for example, a special supplement—usually published by an external company which needs to recoup their costs. You may receive enquiries from the advertising departments, and you may receive enquiries from editorial—very seldom will these two communicate with each other. And rightly so.

> *Remember: In PR you do not have control over the finished product. Too OCD to 'let go'? Book an advert!*

4 Reactive PR

Although there are dozens if not hundreds of ways to end up engaging with the media, all contact mainly boils down to two avenues: reactive, or proactive press relations.

Reactive (involves)

- Providing comment or expertise that's been requested, usually on something topical or in the news.
- Having to speak about, or present a high-profile case or development.

This simply involves 'reacting' to something that is currently happening, either in the industry, world/local news or just a piece that a journalist happens to be working on. It may not necessarily involve a theme that you even want to discuss, consider relevant or which is even your specialty. Reactive media involvement occurs when you, as an expert, are put forward to comment on a topical subject—say, the PIP implant crisis, a rise in men using Botox, or the risks of cosmetic surgery tourism.

On a daily basis, I receive scores of media enquiries asking for expert comment or cosmetic surgery case studies. The following examples are ALL GENUINE.

A freelance journalist is looking for case studies of patients who have undergone cosmetic surgery for a particular reason or landmark occasion—not just for increased self-confidence or health/psychological benefits—for an upcoming story. She is looking specifically for case studies where

- A patient has had pre-wedding plastic surgery.
- A patient has had plastic surgery to boost their career (not modelling).
- Men who have had cosmetic surgery—the journalist would need to speak to their wife/girlfriend.
- Women who have had cosmetic surgery (not a breast augmentation) to help them get over a break up.

The outlet would require pictures and a brief outline of the study as well as to speak to the patient directly.

A production company is working on a 90-minute documentary. The film will follow a diverse group of young people, aged 16–25, who are all unhappy with their appearance, and are planning to make a change. Over the course of 3–6 months the subjects will record their own stories of transformation—from fitness regimes and minor makeovers, to non-surgical treatments and cosmetic surgery—in a video diary format. The subjects may want to record segments of their initial and/or subsequent consultations with a surgeon/in a clinic and their personal feelings about the whole experience. The documentary is in the early stages of production but the producers are hoping to find patients preparing to have cosmetic/reconstructive surgery in the next 3–4 months, who might like to share their stories. They are looking for patients aged 18–25 preparing to undergo any surgical or non-surgical treatments for either medical or cosmetic reasons.

I am looking—urgently—for a woman who says Botox cured her depression. Scientists believe emotions can be 'reverse engineered'—if a patient is prevented from frowning, the theory goes, their brain may think there is nothing to worry about. I am looking for a woman who honestly believes that was the case for her—perhaps she didn't have it done to cure her blues but actually that's what it has done.

I recently read a short piece about 'Collagen marshmallows', available from a department store and was wondering if experts had any stance on whether collagen delivered to the body via food could actually have any anti-aging benefits? Conversely, could there be any potential risks of eating a food that contains collagen?

EXTREME PARTY SEASON COSMETIC SURGERY

Forget breast implants, Botox or tummy tucks. I am looking for women who have had cosmetic surgery in following areas:

1. A 'Toe tuck' where by her toes shortened, or even removed to fit killer heels.
2. Lipo on their 'cankles' (area of leg where the ankle and the calf appear seamless).
3. Removal of bridesmaid bulge (podgy bit between breast and arm pit) for a wedding or night out.

Of course, some of them are more mind-boggling than others …

I am currently writing a story on a trend in America for people to have plastic surgery after they have died to ensure they look good at their funeral.

I'm looking for someone who's had more than 30 cosmetic procedures.

I'm looking for a case study for a feature we're doing about women who have surgery to look like their favourite celebrities. For example, a woman who had lip implants to have lips like Angelina Jolie.

In a nutshell, it is known as 'reactive' PR because you are reacting to an enquiry, to the media's needs. They decide what they want to cover, you just have to be ready for them and make yourself available. Aside from the quirky case study hunting, there are myriad opportunities that would require comment from a cosmetic doctor, surgeon, dermatologist or other clinicians and professionals: from the 10th Anniversary of Botox and the 50th Anniversary of silicone implants, there is a constant stream of relevant news being reported that could be an opportunity for you to impart your knowledge and expertise.

Alternatively, you may be forced to communicate with the press because of involvement with a high-profile case: perhaps using groundbreaking, cutting-edge technology or performing aesthetic treatments on a celebrity. Perhaps it was an unfavourable outcome. In many instances, you may not even welcome the attention—but it's essential that you know how to deal with the media just in case.

Case study I: Ear Implant

I was recently asked to attend a meeting with a Venture Capitalist (VC), funding the work of a surgeon developing a new kind of cosmetic implant currently undergoing clinical trials. The executive began by stating categorically that the surgeon simply wanted to work quietly on his clinical trial, and not be bothered with anything having to do with the press.

Unfortunately, science does not develop in a vacuum and the eyes of the world are always upon developments. In this specific instance, the hospital where the new implant would be offered would be posting information on its website and begin marketing—it had not occurred to the surgeon or their VC that journalists may well find out about the treatment and wish to write about it. They assumed the story wouldn't get out if they didn't proactively seek to put out a press release themselves.

News has a way of getting out, whether you want it or not. Unless you intend to physically gag every patient being treated with some new technique, make no mistake: they will talk to other people, they will blog, they will meet a journalist at a dinner party. You can either choose to manage this process, or as the marketing adage goes, let your public and competitors do it for you.

When I suggested the *Sunday Times* or the *Daily Mail* as potential candidates for an exclusive, the executive sheepishly admitted they had both already been in touch as they had heard though the grapevine (probably through the hospital's PR!) that exciting developments were afoot.

You cannot 'gag' the press for your convenience.

Every time there is news, whether it be of the fluffier variety (reality TV star gets new boobs) or of the more serious kind (cosmetic injectable is taken off the market), as medical professionals you have to be aware that the public is always watching and this represents an opportunity for you. Whether you think it's any of their business or not, they're interested in your views and they want to know what the latest developments are in your practice. So you can make the decision to choose specific outlets to carry your message in a sensible way, or risk it getting out, as it undoubtedly will, losing all control over what is said. Found out about something interesting in the sector? Contact your friendly local journalist—chances are they might not have heard about it: they'll be grateful AND need your expert comment. Win/Win.

Consider 'breaking' news: if you're the first to deliver a story to a journalist, you can ensure that your views are included. Also it fosters a relationship, which means they can remain involved throughout a project or timeframe and cover developments as they happen.

In the case of this new surgical implant, the VC left hurriedly to speak to the surgeon about the importance of negotiating own-ership of media communications. As much as he may have liked to work quietly away in his isolated nerd lab, in the age of 24-hour news channels and the Internet, there are no under-ground bunkers to hide from the prying eyes of the press. News is at a premium.

Case study II: PR Blunder

On a Sunday morning earlier this year I was suddenly bom-barded by scores of panicked emails by outraged PIP victims, up in arms about a supposed Government 'cover-up'. Social media was on fire, with affected women posting on Facebook and Tweeting a shocking U.K. newspaper headline. The story claimed there were results from testing the gel within the con-troversial devices that were being kept 'secret'—that the jour-nalist had tried to secure the study but had been blocked by a government agency.

Whilst answering as many of their frenzied queries as possible, I had to admit I couldn't fathom what the newspaper could possibly be referring to. I was aware of test results from the EU but they were made public and had been available online for weeks. I contacted the newspaper, but as it was a Sunday, the journalist wasn't there. The piece quoted a government agency which had refused to give the information.

By now, law firms smelled blood and hit the media both offline and online with a vengeance, calling publicly for these documents to be released. If the results were so incendiary they were being kept 'secret', WHAT COULD BE IN THEM!!??

I left a voicemail with the newspaper, and rang the governmental agency time and again. It took their Press Officer over 4 hours to get back to me. She seemed confused as to what the fuss was all about—she hadn't even seen any headlines.

First mistake: ALWAYS monitor your press coverage. Even on weekends and holidays, I drive my family mad by checking the media clippings first thing in the morning. I just can't relax until I know there's nothing that could affect any of my clients! The press never sleeps …

I asked if she remembered an interview with this newspaper, and were they by any chance referring to test results that were freely available on the Internet? The Press Officer said vaguely that yes, she did remember a request from a tabloid journalist, but that the document was "over 80 pages long and in medical terminology which their readers probably wouldn't have understood, so I didn't give it to them."

HUGE second mistake: Never patronise the media or the public. Whether you think they have the capabilities to understand something or not, it is not up to you to decide.

It's the journalist's job to translate scientific information into laymen's terms. In the case of negative or controversial news, there's no putting the toothpaste back into the tube. Face issues squarely and as truthfully as possible (see chapter 10 for 'Interview Techniques' and 'Dealing with Difficult Questions').

In this instance it caused hundreds, if not thousands of already worried women, further distress and fostered even more mistrust.

Why would you want to foster close relations with journalists? A lot of the time doctors wonder why the media don't come knocking more often. "But I'm the foremost expert in this area," they declare in shocked, hurt accents. "Why use that *baboon?*" So, why aren't they beating a path to your door?

Journalists have a wide network of experts and publicists that they contact when they're working on a story. Like most people, they'll ring those who they like the best—the friendliest, the ones they've known the longest, or even the one who is most likely to give them what they want. For example, many outlets won't come to me when they need comment on whether this or that celebrity had this or that done. This is simply down to the fact that for the last decade the great majority of my clients have chosen, for their own reasons, not to comment on this sort of thing (as a publicist, I am only the messenger. I cannot influence my clients' behaviour as much as I'd like to sometimes!). So they don't bother. Many of my clients won't agree with a statement they feel is untrue, just for the sake of getting their name in the paper. The media have a name for those experts, they're cheerfully referred to as 'Rent-A-Quotes'.

Clarke's 4th Law: For every expert there is an equal and opposite expert! (known in the legal world as Gibson's Law: for every PhD there is an equal and opposite PhD).

Case study III: Teen Surgery

For years in the U.K., there were surveys being published in teen magazines claiming that 'more and more' teenagers wanted or were undergoing cosmetic surgery. At the time, this simply wasn't the case, but a determined journalist may not always let the truth (as they say) get in the way of a good story.

"Is it true that TENS OF THOUSANDS of girls as young as sixteen are getting nose jobs and boob jobs all around the country?" they demanded on a regular basis. Usually whenever there was a lull in the news, they became desperate to give their editors something juicy.

"No," I would intone wearily. "Our internal polls don't show this. It may well be true that girls are talking about this in schools, but at this time it's not translating to an increase in them actually undergoing surgery."

This will not deter them in many cases, and they will continue the hunt until they find an expert who will endorse their premise that absolutely, their clinics are swamped with dysmorphic teens.

Rent-a-Quote: An expert who will pretty much say or agree to anything on any subject, just to get in the press

Getting on journalists' lists of preferred contacts—resulting in a lot of 'reactive' PR opportunities and therefore coverage—is not achieved by sitting back and letting them find a way to you. It involves hard graft, and not for nothing are there thousands of PR agencies claiming to specialise in the cosmetic surgery sector. Because it takes a lot of time and effort that most doctors and surgeons simply do not have, and also requires a publicist's uniquely honed talents and nose for a good story. Proactive PR results in Reactive PR, the opportunities work symbiotically.

Contacting journalists, asking what they're working on, complimenting them on what they've recently written, helping them with research, providing them with answers that may not even result in coverage for clients but will earn their gratitude—it's an art. Publicists have to walk a fine line between harassing the media, and discreetly making sure their clients are the first choice for anything relevant in their sector. It takes real talent and communication skills, especially when you have something controversial to impart and you choose one outlet over another. Maintaining long-term relationships with hundreds of effectively competing entities all vying for the Next Big Thing requires serious diplomatic abilities and an unflappable temperament. Choose your PR wisely!

Some agencies may defensively insist to their clients they're being 'selective' with what media opportunities they go for, or that it's normal to have very quiet periods for a very long time. But bottom line is, either you have an ongoing, productive relationship with the press or you don't. Organisations with good PR are easy to spot.

I think I'm at my most proud when organisations I represent are mentioned conversationally by famous DJs on the radio, presenters on late-night talk shows and once, a client's name even turned out to be the answer to a famous TV trivia competition. It means that they have a secure place in the public consciousness. When I heard a group of girls in a nightclub chatting about cosmetic surgery and one quoted one of our press articles, I nearly reached over to hug them—which would've been weird, I suppose. But they heard my client was good in bed, so to speak: behold the power of branding!

So at some point you might be tired of having to talk about whatever the press feel is most relevant. Perhaps *you'd* like to call the shots sometime, and establish what the public should be aware of. This is proactive PR.

5 Proactive PR

In this instance, YOU decide what you'd like to speak to the press about. This will involve pursuit on your (or your publicist's) part to:

- Foster relationships with writers and editors
- Share relevant announcements with journalists
- Place you as a 'resident expert'

So how to be proactive and let yourself be known by the media? How to burst onto the media scene? First, you must have something to say that is of importance, and something which you are ideally placed to discuss. That there is something to announce—depending on what this is, it will determine what media (if any) will be interested. For example, company news such as launches and partnerships, new team additions, new services are generally of interest only to the local media. Otherwise, you can find yourself in a situation a little bit like p*ssing down your own leg: it feels really hot to you but not to anyone else!

In health care specifically, I have found a 'Golden Triangle' of themes that will almost always guarantee you media coverage:

- New procedures, techniques or technology
- Statistics and trends
- Human interest

We'll go into further detail as to how to pitch to journalists in a further chapter, but first we need to determine what actually makes—and what doesn't make—a newsworthy announcement.

But suffice to say that proactive PR is the basis of all successful media relations. It starts with you, and inasmuch as is possible with the press, you call the shots. However, it is worth reiterating the difference between PR and advertising outlined in chapter 3: you will never be able to control everything that the journalist puts into the article or piece, and this is why it is called *editorial*. If you want to establish the column width, who else is quoted and how it is edited, book an advert!

CONTROLLING COPY

Journalists don't tell you how to perform procedures, and many will find it frankly insulting when you demand to approve their copy. It is very rare that this is ever an option—and it drives the majority of them crazy when experts ask for this. Most concede to doing a 'read back' to case studies, because they understand that patients feel vulnerable and at times is the only way that they will secure their participation. There are certain exceptions—by now a great number of journalists know, and trust, me well enough to occasionally run their copy past me if we're covering something contentious. But this is because they're safe in the knowledge that I will only check for accuracy, and leave their writing, tone and general gist unmolested. Should I start pointing out style suggestions, or criticising other experts they've chosen to include, they won't let me look next time.

A NOTE ON OTHER 'EXPERTS'

I've had clients grumble that other experts are also included in the piece. You need to know that neither you nor I have any authority over who else is included, and many times journalists have to include more than one voice. For example, if a new procedure or technique is launched, with claims of wonderful amazingness never seen before, the writer of this piece (if worth their salt), will need to seek an independent opinion. Whether there ever is such a thing may be up to question, but the reality is they cannot (or shouldn't) run a one-sided piece. This is, again, what advertising is for. Thus, do not get cheesed off when you launch THE BEST FACELIFT TECHNIQUE THAT EVER WAS, and some random doctor (to whom you probably taught EVERYTHING THEY KNOW) says it's a bit Meh. Journalists have to get a second opinion. Don't want anyone dissing your stuff? Once again I suggest you look into booking an advert as per chapter 3.

COURTING CONTROVERSY

CASE STUDY: 'Any publicity is good publicity'

I remember early in my career there was a cosmetic surgery provider that would launch ever more outrageous promotional gimmicks. Without fail, each time they provided the press release as an 'exclusive' to a journalist who knew me well. Inevitably, she would ask my clients for an opinion, which they would do willingly, and scathingly. It took us all, including the journalist, a while to catch on that they were actually doing it on purpose. In a 'any publicity is good publicity' approach, they had decided that they would actually generate more column inches by being criticised, than by simply being mentioned in one sympathetic article that would be lost as tomorrow's chip paper. Instead, the outrage and controversy surrounding their offers would burn for days, giving them exposure that money couldn't buy. In effect, they were 'trolling' for press coverage!

Tips: Courting controversy can be an effective way of achieving exposure—but whether you're engaging in off-the-wall stunts or 'naming and shaming' bad practice, ensure that you're acting in line with your brand, ethos and the image you wish to project.

If you take away one message from a proactive PR, take this: it involves time, and effort. I get approached a lot for 'mini-campaigns': let's PR me/my clinic for a month, or 3 months. See what happens. There is no way you can ever appropriately, fully gauge the success of a PR campaign in that period of time. First off, monthly magazines have a 4-month lead time. If you want to be in *Cosmopolitan, Glamour, Harper's Bazaar* and *Tatler*, I could potentially place you tomorrow and you won't see an article until well into the next season. Want to know EXACTLY when the piece is due to come out? Once again, refer to chapter 3 and book and advert! I've started work with new clients who, after 6 weeks, compare themselves with clients that have had PR continuously for 6, 7, even 9 years. That kind of coverage takes ages to achieve and you have to trust the process …

> *Remember to treat your PR agency like you would a gym or health club membership: paying a fee every month isn't automatically going to do anything for you. Invest time in the relationship, invest the effort. The best publicist cannot make something out of nothing.*

The media have a really bad habit of thinking you've gone out of business if they don't hear from you in a while. They will not track you down, to find out whether this is the case or not. From a business perspective, I have to take on short-term projects. Sometimes the client just has one product launch or one announcement to make, and we all have to pay our bills. But Rome wasn't built in a day and a secure place in the consumer mind is not achieved in 3–6 months. It may well be that during that period your PR agency works hard at fostering awareness among the press about you, and only on the fourth month does the journalist decide "OK, I'm ready to do a feature about this." It's a shame if the PR's answer has to be "Well, we don't work with them anymore. BUT we work with this other guy/clinic/product …!"

Because, don't kid yourselves. You're great, but PR agents don't pass on media leads out of the goodness of their hearts. The only way we can live with the levels of stress involved in protecting and enhancing dozens, if not hundreds, of people and companies' reputations, is by knowing that we are providing a service that is remunerated fairly. Thus, when you cancel a PR contract, and suggest jocularly "keep sending me anything relevant!" be aware that your agency's "sure we will" is 100% sarcastic and subtexted with IN YOUR DREAMS. Media opportunities don't grow on trees, they are jealously guarded and cherished and with extremely rare exceptions, rightly passed onto the people that pay for them.

> *PR is not a right you've earned by your sheer awesomeness (a quality that we do not dispute, mind).*

To really delve into 'proactive' PR, first we have to examine what the press would consider worth their time …

6 What is newsworthy?

By and large, the great majority of clients I have dealt with over the years have all wanted to feature prominently in the consumer press, rather than the industry media. There is of course a trade element that can be sought—magazines and websites aimed specifically at peers in the 'industry', but mostly they know that in a sea of choice, their prospects have to make a decision and the public relies heavily on the media to help them in their quest. Just like we all do when choosing things like breakfast cereal and running shoes, whether consciously or unconsciously, we retain scraps of information from articles we've read and radio programmes we listened to.

What isn't newsworthy—or, Like p*ssing down your leg (feels hot to you but not to anyone else)

- Refurbishing your office: I had a client once who kept insisting on having a press event, because they'd bought new sofas from Italy for their waiting room. Hey editors, hold the front page!
- You've started offering cosmetic injectables. Yep, you and everyone else.
- You have an AMAZING case study, but no 'before' photos.
- You have an AMAZING case study, but the photos are crap.
- You have an AMAZING case study, but they refuse to be identified.
- Having polled your patients, you found that 95% care about their appearance: well, yes, they're in your office to begin with …
- Having polled your patients, you find that men worry about losing their hair. Whoop-de-do.
- Piggybacking on a current trend which makes no sense: there was a lot in the news about bullying, and one client—a very well respected physician—asked whether we could do a story about the

fact he'd been bullied for a year when he was 9. I asked if this had been instrumental in his career success. "Not really," he shrugged.

- You claim there's a rise in a certain type of patient, but can't back this up with a case study or any statistics.
- You claim the procedures you perform change lives, but no one will come forward to illustrate this.
- You have a new secretary/receptionist/cleaner.

Journalists receive literally thousands of press releases every day. What news do you have to impart that they will find relevant? I refer back to the 'Golden Triangle' of cosmetic surgery PR:

- New procedures or techniques
- Studies and statistics
- Human interest

These are not by any means the ONLY themes that should be explored, but in my experience they are the closest to a 'sure thing' in terms of securing coverage. Other areas include partnership announcements, new team additions, involvement with the local community (such as charity endeavours) and hometowners. I will go into these in further detail, but one extra dimension that is worth noting (and could arguably make the 'Golden Triangle' into a 'Golden Square') is the bonus element: Celebrity!

Nothing enthuses the media more than a notable, no matter how vague their claim to fame, admitting they've had this or that done. Because it's so rare that bona fide famous people (generally Hollywood actors or well-known artists) ever admit to having aesthetic treatments, finding these B–Z list celebs can be a gold mine. But like everything in Marketing, it has to be weighed against your brand. Is your clinic Jersey/Geordie Shore or is it Made in Chelsea/Housewives of Beverly Hills? Keep in mind that celebs do garner column inches, but you also want them to be a good ambassador for you. Also be aware that, for the most part, they expect greatly discounted—if not outright free—treatment.

> *Remember that having a well-known patient can also backfire—should (God forbid) anything go wrong, it will also be happening in the public eye.*

Even when you're referring to an established or well-known procedure, having an updated 'tweak' or slightly changed aspect can automatically make it newsworthy. It could be given a unique name that appeals to the public (the 'Madonna lift', the Brazilian Tummy Tuck, the 'Pippa bottom' ...), or it could be based on an article recently accepted in a medical journal, which automatically lifts it to a more credible level in the eyes of serious journalists.

EXAMPLES

THE INNOVATIVE TECHNIQUE THAT HAS THEM IN STITCHES

He Sutures, He Scores: An Expert Presents Modified Technique to Prevent Ear Loss

A leading plastic surgeon and world expert on ear reconstruction has devised an innovative, modified otoplasty (pinning back prominent ears) procedure that could prevent problems such as ear deformity or loss by using stitches, instead of the commonly used technique of scoring. He presented his modification to this underused technique at the Academic Conference on Otolaryngology—the main event for head and neck surgeons and allied health professionals.

Previously, techniques involving sutures (stitches) had always been deemed safer but less permanent, because the sutures could 'cheesewire' through the cartilage and allow the ear to stick out again. To combat this, the surgeon developed an unusual modification using a 'fascial flap'—an extra layer of tissue taken from the tough covering under the skin on the side of the head. This protects the more delicate tissues, holds the sutures firm and prevents them from cutting through.

Says Dr. X:

"For many years, the accepted technique for otoplasties has been anterior scoring. The skin of the back surface of the ear is stripped off the cartilage and then the cartilage is scored (as you would

do the fat on a piece of pork) to weaken it. However, I came to realise that most of the problematic, legal cases I came across throughout my career had used this technique and in almost all cases of ear loss and deformity, the cause was an infected haematoma—a pool of blood which slowly developed within the ear after surgery."

Another advantage of this technique is that patients can precisely stipulate just how far they would prefer their ears to stick out. The accepted norm tends to be 19 mm, but some patients insist on a more 'tucked-in', 'slicked-back' look. This technique also avoids the characteristic 'telephone deformity'—so called because the middle part of the ear can end up closer to the head than the rest of the ear.

New French Lip Procedure Lets You Bin the Lip Gloss

(Or, 'Why French Women Don't Have Trout Pouts')

A quick, painless and subtle lip enhancement procedure that can be done in your lunch hour, which will give you perfect 'bee-stung' lips has been launched by a top French cosmetic doctor. Dr. X developed and honed his technique over the years in Paris, as he was appalled at the overtly obvious filler treatments he witnessed in magazines and television.

The 'French Lip', or 'non-volume' enhancement procedure involves injecting a hyaluronic acid solution into the lips using very small pin-prick injections around the lip line and only on the top layer of the lip rather than the muscle. It takes around half an hour to complete and the result is naturally shiny, subtly 'plumped' lips, which will last from 6 months to a year, depending on the patient.

According to area patient Y:

"The procedure was painless and the result is fantastic. I have always had quite thin lips and now I have a lovely dewy pout that exactly suit my face and dimensions. It looks so natural I can finally throw away the lip gloss!"

The hyaluronic acid solution is injected into the 'red' top layer of the lips just under the skin and not into the muscle, as traditionally done in lip-enhancement treatments. This gives what the doctor refers to as a subtle 're-plumping' effect without actually adding volume. Because the solution hydrates the lips, it also leaves them shiny and glossy.

Should a patient feel their lips are slightly more plumper than they envisioned, there is even an antidote so they can be reduced.

Dr. X said:

"Patients are safe in the knowledge that the substance injected is one that naturally occurs in their body and if for any reason they wanted their lips reduced we could reverse it immediately. But we haven't had to do that yet, as we always aim for a very subtle look."

A CHECKLIST

- Is the procedure new, or does it have a new 'tweak' or edge?
- If it's published in a journal, or presented at a conference/symposium include a link to this.
- Ideally you will have a case study to illustrate the procedure (more on that later), but if there aren't any photos, diagrams can also work. It's important to make the story 'visual' in some way.
- Include quotes on why this development is of importance to the profession or the public, and outline its benefits.
- Make sure it is written in laymen terms.

STUDIES, STATISTICS AND TRENDS

The press cannot get enough of these, and relevant statistics will be re-used over and over, providing continuous, ongoing coverage. What's harder sometimes is pinpointing what the media will find of interest. If a poll, it should be questions that haven't been asked before or are phrased in such a way that they can provide headline-grabbing fodder. Studies and statistics can vary widely from the serious to the trivial (which makes it no less interesting to the press). An article in a medical journal about advances in fat transfer to the breast is as interesting to the media as a poll regarding the 'best celebrity buttocks'. All that varies is the outlet that you will be pitching this to, which we will cover in another chapter.

Trends are fascinating and what you notice in your own practice—say, a rise in a particular demographic or profession—may well be considered of relevance by the press and in particular anything specific to your geographic area. Are you seeing more baby boomers? Are you noticing stressed-out bankers clamouring for Botox to keep a 'poker face' in the boardroom? A rise in teachers having treatments in the summer so they can recuperate away from prying schoolchildren? Is there a spate of patients in the New Year, eager to spend their holiday gift money? Are people turning away from a certain type of treatment in favour of another? What are the reasons for this? All of these are matters of interest to the press.

EXAMPLES

ALL YOU NEED IS LIPO: BOOMERS DOMINATE LOCAL COSMETIC SURGERY

Leading Cosmetic Surgeon Reveals Local Age Trends

Area baby boomers in their race to stay young looking are increasingly turning to cosmetic surgery as an anti-aging weapon, according to leading local cosmetic surgeon X, where more than one in three patients at her clinic are now in their 50s and 60s.

Area patient Y, aged 62, says she has found confidence and a new lease of life after having liposuction to her inner thighs, back, hips and stomach.

She says:

"I have always been fairly fit and my shape has remained the same—but I hit a stage where I suddenly gained weight and no amount of diet or exercise would shift it. I've always been a gym goer and had never experienced this before, so was quite alarmed. Clothes shopping became a nightmare and I'd come home feeling deflated—nothing seemed to fit or look right—it really affected my confidence. I decided the only route was cosmetic surgery. Once I'd made the decision to have liposuction I booked in immediately. The procedure was a lot more comfortable than I expected and was pleasantly surprised by how I felt afterwards. When I looked at the instant new shape I had I was delighted."

Baby boomers is a term generally applied to adults in their 50s and 60s, and they are the leading group opting to spend their disposable cash on making themselves look and feel good.

According to the surgeon:

"Baby boomers are fuelling the surge for cosmetic procedures. They are more focused on themselves, they work to stay fit and healthy and as a result want to look younger. Boomers have seen their offspring fly the nest and now see it as 'their turn' to invest in themselves and take time out to make sure they look and feel their best. Some are doing it because they generally want to look younger, and can finally afford it. Others may be starting over again after a life-changing event, such as divorce or illness."

NINE OUT OF TEN WOMEN WANT A BOOB JOB, A THIRD SAY HUBBY WILL PAY

New Survey by Cosmetic Surgery Chat Show Reveals Nation's Wants

New figures released today reveal that although over half of women (55%) wish to alter the size/shape of their breasts, a whopping 9 out of 10 (89%) want a non-surgical option such as the 'boob jab', despite publicized concerns about injections in the breast area.

The survey, undertaken to mark the debut of the nation's first-ever 'myth-busting' cosmetic surgery TV chat show, also found that women weren't entirely alone in their desire for enhanced breasts, with nearly a quarter (23%) of men saying they actually prefer 'fake' breasts. The survey also revealed the public's favourite celeb breasts!

The groundbreaking, independent programme will review these results, interview some of the most well-respected surgeons and also tackle some of the most common misconceptions about cosmetic surgery, including the myth that implants burst at high altitudes.

Survey highlights

- Over half (55%) of women said the first thing they would change, given the chance, would be the size of their breasts, with more than two out of five (42%) saying liposuction to reduce tummy fat would come first.
- Nearly three out of five (63%) women said their main concern about having breast implants is that their breasts would look fake, so would prefer methods of enhancement which can give more natural results.
- A third (33%) of women said their partner/spouse would be happy to pay for their breast surgery.
- Nearly half (47%) of women think, incorrectly, that breast implants can burst at high altitudes.
- Nearly a quarter of men (23%) actually prefer surgically enhanced breasts, while two out of five (40%) said it didn't bother them.
- When asked to name the first one cosmetic surgery procedure that popped into their heads, 71% said breast surgery with 18% mentioning liposuction.

The survey was carried out among 523 people in Manchester and London during February 2010, using web surveys and on-street interviews.

A CHECKLIST FOR YOUR TRENDS PIECE

- Have you identified an original trend, perhaps one that bucks expectations? For example, if annual statistics are released in your sector, does your practice/hospital/region corroborate or even surpass these?
- Back your premise with figures whenever possible: a percentage or numbers rise, but be careful with these—most journalists nowadays will query a '500% change' and assume you mean five patients.
- Make sure you have an example—ideally a fully identifiable case study—that exemplifies this trend.
- Think visually. Is it an original area of the body or demographic that the journalist can illustrate.
- ALWAYS posit a theory or explanation for the trend: a rise in men having tummy tucks (post-obesity) or women seeking buttock enhancement (Hip-Hop/Latin culture …). You can't just say 'patients are getting younger' without explaining why!
- Make it interesting or witty.

If I had to pinpoint one area that is almost guaranteed to garner interest from the press, I would say that this is it—the main area you should focus on the most. Having a patient willing to share their experience with the world is invaluable. There is no point in saying that 70 year olds are having more lip fillers, or 50-year-old men are having chemical peels or gynaecomastia ops if you don't have someone that will actually back up/illustrate this claim.

In cosmetic surgery there is usually a dearth of willing case studies, mainly because many patients don't want their friends and family—let alone their neighbours or work colleagues—to know that they've undergone any procedures. Also, with time the requirements of the press have become more and more exacting: they no longer want just someone who had a nose job, they want someone whose life has been *transformed* by their nose job.

One thing that is worth noting is that sometimes, the patient you are absolutely sure would rather gouge his/her own eyes out than appear in the press talking about their flabby belly or bingo wings can sometimes completely surprise you with their willingness to go public. And equally, the most extroverted patients who shout from the rooftops that they've had their square jaw softened by fillers and Botox treatment may suddenly shy away from actually speaking about it to a reporter. It is important that in this, the most essential area of your PR, you have the commitment from your team to help you secure and collate a wide range of ideal cases.

HOW TO SPOT A CASE STUDY

There is often confusion surrounding the difference between 'testimonials' and case studies for PR; what they are and what is expected of them. Here we aim to clarify and define this by giving tips on how to spot a good case study and outlining the process so there is no ambiguity about the extent of their involvement.

Case studies versus testimonials

Case studies are patients who are happy to have their story and accompanying photographs featured in the media. In nearly all instances, they will be required to be fully identified, that is, show their faces. It is extremely rare that they will be allowed to remain anonymous, although they may be able to change their names (so press coverage doesn't appear on Google if someone looks them up, for example).

Testimonials are usually quotes from patients that are featured on a clinic's website or marketing materials, giving their recommendation on the treatment/service, for the benefit of potential patients. Sometimes when patients are asked to be case studies, they assume this is what is required of them and are horrified when they're asked to appear on a TV show and talk about their acne.

What we require from a PR perspective are the former, that is, *case studies*.

Sourcing case studies

The clinician/practitioner will be able to use their judgement as to whether to ask a patient if they'd be willing to participate in publicity for the clinic. It is often the case that it is their nurse or even receptionist who picks up on the good stories when chatting to patients in a more informal way than the actual clinician, so it is important that all staff members are fully briefed to keep an eye out. Gently probing questions can be worked into conversation, such as asking the patients why they are having treatment, or why now? There could be a variety of interesting stories lurking behind their decision such as how they're funding the procedure—perhaps they won the lottery or had an inheritance or divorce payout. Perhaps they have a unique motivation: a wedding, starting to date again … you won't know unless you ask.

> *The most newsworthy human interest story could be sitting in your waiting room right now!*

What makes a good case study?

The following information will enable you to help the patients make an informed decision. If a patient is still not clear/sure, it is always best to obtain their consent for their number to be passed to the PR handler to call and talk through the process in a sensitive manner.

- Patients who have had a brand new procedure, which may be known to the profession, but has not been widely publicised in consumer media outlets.
- Even if the results aren't dramatic or the procedure isn't new, the patients may have an interesting story to tell—perhaps their treatment helped them to get over an emotional barrier, made them feel more confident, made them feel years younger, etc. Maybe their treatment was inspired by a friend/relative/partner having treatment, or maybe the catalyst was a special event such as an upcoming wedding, gift money.
- The patient ideally needs to be able to demonstrate a notable visible difference or change—the more dramatic the better. Strong before-and-after photos are essential! Occasionally, the patients don't like the clinical photos, but have their own candid shots that can demonstrate the difference.
- The patient needs to be comfortable with being initially interviewed by the PR handler and, if there is media interest in the story, also by a journalist (usually just telephone interview suffices, unless there is TV involved).
- The patient needs to be willing to disclose photographs—including their face.

Please note

Patients must be emotionally strong enough to answer press questions. Although not usually inappropriately probing, it might not be ideal for someone who is feeling too 'raw' after a bereavement or significant life change.

Publicists are not (normally) looking to be flippant about any case study story!! Each one is generally treated with respect and in a highly professional manner, or at least, they are by my team. The case studies are used to highlight the skills of the clinician or the excellent results of a particular treatment. Publicists can offer some basic media training to them, or a mock interview, if participants are unsure about the process.

Photography

For any case studies we will need clear before and after photos in high resolution (usually the 'best' setting on a digital camera), so they can be reproduced at good quality in a publication. Journalists are looking for case studies that show as dramatic a difference as possible.

Some magazines and newspapers prefer to do their own photo shoots. These are normally scheduled around the patient's diary and a photographer may visit the case studies at their home. If they are required to attend a studio, magazines will generally reimburse travel expenses.

A good way to obtain high-quality photography and motivate patients to take part in publicity is to offer a professional photo shoot, with the patient getting a set of prints in return for allowing the shots to be used publicly.

Payment for stories

Some magazines pay case studies for their stories and will require the patient to sign exclusivity agreements. Payments can vary widely, depending on the strength of the personal story.

Some clinics like to offer certain patients a discount or 'freebie' as a thank you.

Interviews

Requests for interviews by journalists should be checked for suitability, and whether they 'match' the organisation's brand and target market. Traditionally, your publicist will then call the patient to gain their consent to pass on contact details and guide the patient through the process. It is my own agency's practice never to pass on contact details of patients to journalists without permission, but preferably allow them to make contact of their own volition and from a private number should they so wish.

Consumer versus professional/trade press

Case studies are of interest to both consumer and trade press. The trade press is usually interested in the overview of the treatment and the visible outcome—that is, clinical before and afters. They are not usually interested in the patient's personal 'journey'. Consumer press, however, will always be interested in the 'real-life' aspects of the story.

Consent

It is usually the responsibility of the clinic/practitioner to gain consent from the patient to take part in publicity. Sometimes, after agreeing to take part, patients can have second thoughts, occasionally after discussing it with their partner, spouse or even children. Needless to say, you should never put them under any pressure to continue with the story if they are uncomfortable. It is a good idea to have a standard form to ask them to sign in advance, stating they have agreed to take part in press articles and have photographs issued, to ensure there is no ambiguity surrounding their involvement.

Patients are generally thrilled when the story comes out and keep the articles as a nice memento.

EXAMPLES (all genuine—names have been changed)

NOT SO NOSEY ANYMORE

Non-Surgical Nose Job for Jonathan

Since breaking his nose at the age of 14 playing baseball at school, Jonathan Smith has suffered from an unsightly bump, changing the shape of his profile and making his nose appear much bigger than it is. Jason, who is now 26 and from the area, had been teased about its shape through his teen years but was always averse to having surgery. Despite nose jobs being the most popular procedure among men, going under the knife seemed extreme to Jason for various reasons including price, the fact the results would be permanent and the length of recovery time—so he was delighted to discover there are less invasive procedures that could emulate the results of a nose job but without the worry of recovery or pain. Jason booked in for his non-surgical treatment with a top aesthetic practitioner and celeb favourite Dr. X, who injected a series of dermal fillers to create a far more streamlined profile.

Says Jonathan:

"I've never liked the bump in the middle of my nose but never wanted to go under the knife as I was conscious the results are permanent, and I know it's an invasive procedure that requires a lot of down time. The procedure with Dr. X took about 20 minutes and didn't hurt in the slightest! I'd spent a few months researching the procedure and researched Dr. X, then booked to go and see him. I am over the moon with the results."

According to Dr. X:

"Jonathan's procedure involved a series of injections with dermal fillers (Restylane) to improve the appearance of his nose and smooth his profile. The whole procedure took just over 20 minutes and the patient was able to continue with his day as normal, with no pain. The procedure is not permanent, however Jonathan is able to continue with the injections as and when he wants them done, giving him the freedom to make the decision around his own schedule, knowing there is minimal risk and no recovery time. It's great to see how delighted he is with the results and how confident he feels now about his appearance."

HANNAH FINALLY GETS HER BOOB JOB—AGED 65!

From OAP to OMG

After 15 years of looking after her critically ill husband and raising their children, a 65-year-old pensioner decided it was high time she invested in herself. When her husband sadly passed away last summer, area woman Hannah Jones, finally took the plunge and got she always wanted: a boob job. The former glamour model opted for a breast enlargement in November of last year—taking her from an A to an F cup to restore her bust to the size it had been before having children.

Says Hannah:

"I used to do modeling so looked after my body and it's paid off over the years as I've maintained a nice, slim shape. However after carrying four children, coupled with getting older, my breast volume decreased and I was very unhappy with them. I always wanted to have a boob job to rectify it but it never seemed to be the right time, and then my husband fell ill and I nursed him through the next 15 years before he sadly passed away last year. I spent so much time looking after him, and the children as they grew up, that I never had the time or energy to invest in doing something like having cosmetic surgery, so it simply fell by the wayside."

"With the children now grown up and my husband now not here I felt it was time to dedicate some time to living my life and I booked in for a breast enlargement in November, after a consultation with local cosmetic surgeon X. He made me feel totally at ease and the op went very well—I couldn't have wished for better treatment or care. I now feel so much more confident about myself and I feel it's actually given me a new lease of life. My children have been very supportive of my decision and can see the difference it's made to me. I'd urge anyone considering cosmetic surgery to go for it—if there's something you're unhappy with why not change it?"

Breast augmentation is still the most popular cosmetic surgery and has risen by more than 10% on the previous year.

The surgeon says:

"I think Hannah's case demonstrates perfectly that it doesn't matter what age you are, cosmetic surgery can dramatically improve your quality of life if there has been something you have been unhappy with about your appearance, and you have the right expectations. Breast augmentation may be a procedure

usually associated with younger women or women in their 30s and 40s who have lost breast volume due to pregnancy and childbirth, but in this case it's achieved great results for this patient. She's happier and more confident as a result and that's what it's all about."

(NB: This press release resulted in at least a dozen extensive features over several months, in many women's magazines, over 50s titles, local radio programmes and national newspapers.)

CHECKLIST

- Have you got an identifiable case study, and do they understand what's required of them?
- Ensure you have good before-and-after photos of any procedures, where you can easily see the difference.
- Include details such as the patient's full name (even if it's a fake one), age, job, marital status and where they live.
- Make sure you explain the procedure involved.
- The press release or case study notes should have information such as when they had the treatment.
- Quotes from the practitioner should be included as well as the patient, who should ideally describe his/her experience and the impact it had on their life.
- Very important: Is the case study available for interviews? There is no point issuing a press release about their treatment if they're about to go on holiday or are under work constraints.

A note on free or discounted treatment in exchange for publicity

Although, as mentioned, there are no guarantees in PR, a good publicist can work on angles and case studies even *before* a patient has undergone any procedures. What we'll tend to do is write the press release as if the treatment has taken place, and we 'shop' this around to likely outlets to gauge interest. This means that the clinic or hospital can then proceed with the discount or freebie, with the peace of mind that there are already journalists who wish to cover the story. I have lost count of the amount of times that new clients or clinicians I have met at conferences have told me that they did this or that procedure for free and never got anything out of it. This way, such a situation can be prevented as much as possible.

Personally, I have no real judgements about free or discounted procedures in exchange for publicity and am aware that this approach may be frowned upon in some quarters; however, this is simply part and parcel of cosmetic surgery PR. In some instances, this will simply be the only way to secure a willing, first-hand account. The majority of people who undergo facelifts and Botox and liposuction do not, as a general rule, want to share their experiences with national newspapers, glossy magazines or morning television. They don't want to show their wrinkled or saggy 'before' photos and this is not to be wondered at. So here I'm just showcasing the options available to you, not necessarily encouraging any practices you don't feel comfortable with.

Tip: Could the patient get anything out of the publicity? Perhaps they've written a book, or own a local salon that could get a mention in the piece ...

Using employees as case studies

Over the years I've seen more volunteer case studies put forward who are employees of the clinic or hospital. This is quite natural—they're a captive audience and more educated about the treatment. In addition, they may be eligible for staff discounts anyways. It has always been my recommendation that you do not hide the fact that they work for you from the journalists in question. It may well be that they ultimately decide against using the case study as some magazines and newspapers have a policy against this sort of thing, because they don't judge the patient story to be entirely impartial; or they might work with you on coming up with the best way of presenting the story—however, it will cost you the relationship if they find out they're being lied to. I find that being honest and genuine helps in the long run, because there is no point hiding that the person works there, which they could find out if they're listed in the staff section of the website, or someone recognises them.

First-hand accounts: journalists as case studies

Some of the most powerful stories, winning hands down, are when journalists themselves undergo a treatment or procedure. They are wordsmiths; they have the ability and power to make it sound like the best decision a person could ever make.

Like in any sector, in journalism there are responsible journalists, and less responsible ones. Some will even refuse free treatment (although this is becoming more rare), because it might impair their ability to report their experience in an unbiased way. I pride myself in having relationships with those that take their cosmetic surgery reporting more seriously, but as mentioned in chapter 3, the thing about editorial is that ultimately it cannot be controlled. Just because a reporter came to your clinic and underwent a procedure, there is no guarantee that they will afterwards rave, or indeed write about it at all. This is why experienced publicists are worth their weight in gold. They can spot an opportunist a mile away. There are, sadly, plenty of them who know that clinics are desperate for press coverage and they negotiate steep discounts for their (or manage to get outright free) procedures and the promised media coverage later on never materialises. I know of clinics and hospitals that offer the discount on the condition of coverage running, and charge the journalist should it not appear. Keep in mind, however, that sometimes the reporter is simply waiting for a chance to run the article and their editors are amenable. Stay in touch with them.

Areas the press can't get enough of—or Lips and Boobs are so passé ...

The media particularly enjoy plastering photos of celebs alongside their stories. It increases the chances that viewers/readers will stick around. Areas around the body they seem to enjoy highlighting are also becoming more unusual:

- Shoulders
- Toes
- Dimples
- Hands
- Man-boobs: in cosmetic surgery PR, this is the gift that keeps on giving
- Buttocks
- Earlobes
- Feet
- Knees

- Genitals (I'm just the messenger …)
- Anything they can give a weird nickname to, for example, cankles (fat calves), bridesmaid's bulge (fatty bit between breast and armpit), bingo wings

OTHER ANGLES

Aside from new procedures and techniques, studies and statistics, and human interest, are there other potential story angles to develop or refine within? We will be exploring in the next chapter how to determine the best audience, but consider your offering and whether there might be any material in:

- Technology: Would technology magazines be interested? Most newspapers will have a journalist that covers this beat.
- Science: As above, there is usually a science desk and also science-focused magazines.
- Health care: Angles consumer empowerment, personal improvement and well-being that are of interest to health care as a whole rather than just aesthetics.
- Business: Have you thought of doing a story about your company, clinic or hospital as a business? Does the product you're launching have an interesting, entrepreneurial story behind it?
- Local: Are you engaging in any particular way with your local community? Consider 'Hometowners'—the local newspapers and radio from where you (or members of your team) grew up may be fascinated by what you're doing. They like their 'local boy/girl done good' stories. Also any involvement with charities—for example, is your entire team taking part in a marathon, or is one of your staff doing anything interesting like a parachute jump (for a good cause, not for Spring Break)? These are all good ways of 'plugging' your name!
- 'Verticals': Is your case study of a particular walk of life that would make their story interesting to the media outlets of their profession? Air stewards, GPs, the military, sportspeople … remember they all have their own magazines and blogs.

7 Knowing your audience (or Don't try and get down wit' da kidz)

- National press versus local/regional
- Trade versus consumer
- Newspapers
- Male/Female lifestyle: demographics
- Consumer Health
- Other specialist magazines
- Broadcast
- Blogs

Of all the steps you need to take to successfully launch and run a Public Relations campaign, it is failing to grasp who your audience is that can cause the most serious problems, and leading to your press announcement falling flat: causing as much impact as a fart in a wind tunnel.

This is an area full of pitfalls—you need to keep in mind not just the outlet you're liaising with, but also the journalist and their specific target audience. Radio stations have completely different targets in terms of demographics. *Cosmopolitan, Grazia, Elle, Glamour* and *Allure* may seem like they're all similar women's titles but they each have different readerships that vary in taste and purchasing behaviour. You will need to keep this in mind both reactively—if they've contacted you for comment—and proactively, when determining what might be likely to secure their attention.

Although national coverage is fantastic for credibility ("as seen in" *USA Today, The Times*), most clients find that actually it is their local press that is most effective in terms of securing enquiries. This is because, although it's not entirely unheard of, it's less likely that someone will travel from Cleveland to New Jersey, or from Newcastle to Bristol for a boob job or some Botox. However, if your news ticks the 'newsworthiness' boxes, you can easily determine whether the story is of national, regional or micro-local importance.

> *Tip: Are you interested in international press? Have you thought of targeting specific airline, train or hotel magazines? Note that this market can be tricky to break and occasionally may expect advertising investment as well. But if it's your target market, go for it! (more on specialist magazines later.)*

The local press can be difficult—believe me, your average Small Town Bugle can be more exacting and sniffy than even the national press. This is because they know how effective it can be for local businesses to achieve coverage and they drive a hard bargain. If they can get you to book an ad instead, they will try! Having said that, there are means of securing their interest and that is by ensuring that your story ticks the boxes of what makes a story 'local'. Involvement with the community always helps—sponsoring or participating in local events, charity awareness days and other opportunities abound. Keep in mind that they are not there to service YOU. Just because you're offering, say, free mole mapping during skin cancer awareness week doesn't automatically mean that the paper considers this to be news. They may expect you to book an ad to promote this—however, if you're able to give them real news in the form of a local patient story or some new statistics, they may consider it worth some editorial.

CASE STUDY: Local

SUPPORT FROM LOCAL CLINIC HAS BUDDING OLYMPIAN JUMPING FOR JOY

Trampoline Gymnast Gets Funds Boost

A budding local Olympic trampoline gymnast is jumping for joy after a local consultancy for cosmetic surgery and aesthetic treatments stepped in with sponsorship to help fund training for the 12-year-old girl. Jane Harrison's dream to represent the country at Olympic level is being supported by local clinic X, the premier destination for all cosmetic surgery procedures in the area.

Jane has been training in trampoline gymnastics from the age of 5 and competing since she was 9 years old. In November, she will compete at National level for her club, the local Trampoline Gymnastics Academy, and she will also compete in the national synchronised trampoline gymnastics competition—which last year saw her achieve second place.

Says Emma's mum Sharon:

"We're absolutely thrilled that the clinic has decided to support Jane's ambitions, in the sport to which she has become extremely dedicated. It is something we have committed to as a family, as the training costs are high and travel to the training involves a 40 mile round trip four times a week. The clinic's sponsorship is gratefully received."

X clinic, located in Y, has funded half of the annual training costs—which amounts to £1,500 (roughly $2,000). Says the plastic surgeon and lead clinician:

"Jane shows great ambition, and according to experts, great talent too. At our clinic we're delighted to help her get one step closer to her Olympic dream via the national competitions. We wish her every success for the future."

(NB: This press release resulted in extensive local media coverage, including a photo op with the plastic surgeon on a trampoline!)

PINK IS THE NEW BLACK THIS HALLOWEEN!

Clinic scrubs up pink to raise money for Breast Cancer Awareness

A local day surgery centre offering the latest treatments in anti-aging, dermatology, cataract, dental and vascular surgery is 'scrubbing up' pink this Halloween to raise awareness and funds for Breast Cancer Care.

All the staff at the clinic, including six nurses, aestheticians, admin team and five doctors will be wearing pink this Friday, 31 October as part of Breast Cancer Care's 'In the Pink' month, and encouraging patients and visitors to donate to the cause.

Clinic director comments:

Forget black and scary—everyone here will be in pink this Halloween and even the surgeons will be wearing pink scrubs and masks."

"We believe it is important to give back to the community in some way and Breast Cancer Care is a fantastic charity. It responds to millions of requests every year for support and information on breast cancer concerns and its services are free.

Throughout October, as part of Breast Cancer Awareness month, Breast Cancer Care has been asking the public to get in the *In the Pink* and raise much needed funds for charity.

Tip: Your Village Herald may not be able to spare a reporter to come to your launch, party or fundraising event—however, they will almost always run a piece afterwards if you provide them with photos! So make sure you take some good snaps ...

TRADE VERSUS CONSUMER

Be aware that health and medical journalists in the consumer press—that is, newspapers, magazines and news programmes—know a *little bit* about *a lot*. This means that the journalist who writes about liposuction and Botox, also writes about bird flu, home births, MRSA and eye transplants. The journalists cover a wide range of issues in the health and medical arenas, and are unlikely (except in certain cases where they have a very specific beat) to have in-depth knowledge about any one area. It tends to surprise doctors during interviews when the reporter asks them very basic questions, but in a way, this is what is required of the consumer press. The assumption has to be that the great majority of their audience do not have a medical degree. It is likely that the person interviewing you wrote an article yesterday about sexually transmitted diseases, and tomorrow covering autistic spectrum disorders. So adhere to the famous KISS principle and *Keep it Simple, Stupid!*

There are few journalists that specialise entirely in one health/medical area, although there are exceptions. Cosmetic surgery can be seen to cross a strange boundary between beauty and health, which is why so many beauty writers—who may cover news ranging from moisturiser launches to lipstick and shampoo—will also be writing about Botox and dermal fillers, all under the premise of 'anti-aging'. Do not be fooled into underestimating them: a lot of these beauty mavens really know their stuff. They've spent hours with dermatologists, they've tested products themselves, know their alpha-hydroxy acids from their Retinols and will prod you with sharp questions. There is a growing number of journalists who report on cosmetic surgery alone (with mixed results), as it's such a fascinating subject to the public.

Unfortunately, not all journalists have the tools or the time to understand the science, and especially when inexperienced, they can be fairly susceptible to hype. This goes back to the pressures of having to produce a good story and not having the ability to scrutinise any data very deeply. Help them feel smart by highlighting the important bits—spell it out!

The consumer press is, for the most part, likely to be friendly. Despite what many fearful physicians may believe, they are not there to 'trip you up' or twist your words. They are not there to make you look bad—they are only there to sell a story. You are not a politician, though there may be just as much fascination with what you do (or more). Make their lives easy, and they will come back to you time and again. Their questions will usually be relatively easy to field.

The trade press, however, is a different story. These are reporters who write for scientific journals, for industry magazines, everyday of their lives. They KNOW their stuff. They are more likely to have a relevant background and a deeper knowledge about the subjects you're covering and therefore can ask much more difficult and technical questions. Clients who panic about an interview with *Cosmopolitan* should really worry more about speaking with *Dermatology Today*.

The major difference that must be taken into account between trade and consumer press when considering where to seek exposure for your news is that the trade will always be interested in the science behind the story. The human interest aspect—the patient's 'journey'—is mostly irrelevant to them. As is, for example, the need for full face photos and the patient's wholehearted declaration that "NOW I AM SO CONFIDENT AND I FOUND A NEW BOYFRIEND." In magazines and websites aimed at your peers, you can use clinical before-and-after photography that doesn't identify the patient. These can sometimes be too stark and scary for your average consumer news stand. In consumer press you almost always will be required to identify them. I don't actually know why sometimes it can be such a problem for practitioners to understand this fact. The mainstream media is aimed at regular people, and they want to know how cosmetic surgery affected the patient, how it made them feel—not just where the incision, laser or syringe goes and at what depth. They want to know what effect it's had on the person's life. I still have conversations with clients where they whine "but what's that got to DO with anything?"

In a nutshell: You want to talk science? Go for a journal. You want to be in GQ or morning talk shows? Get your patients to talk about their feelings and show their wedding/holiday photos.

Once again, demographics vary widely—but as mentioned in chapter 3, magazines have that magical quality of living on forever, in doctor's offices and hair salons everywhere. It is essential, however, that you get to know the outlets and who their audience is. There are weeklies, monthlies, gossip rags and fashion glossies. There are magazines aimed specifically at vegetarians, gay men and teenage girls, older women, post-obesity patients, fitness freaks. If they have somehow managed to survive the current economic downturn (painfully affecting print media), know that they have carved themselves a niche that they will hold onto for dear life.

You don't need to have a degree in media studies to determine what the particular audiences are for any given outlet. Your publicist will know, and you should expect a reasonable brief from them before any interviews. Whilst it's true that if you don't have a PR agency, you may not know that (in the U.K.) *Prima* is aimed at women in their 50s, *Woman & Home* aimed at women in their 40s and so on—but all you have to do is look at the covers on a news stand. Almost without fail, the model or celebrity on the cover will be of the target age for their audience. Whether it's the cast of the *Twilight* movies or Dame Helen Mirren, it will give you a clue as to who they're writing for.

We will go into interview techniques further in this book, but knowing the target demographics of the outlets you're speaking with is as essential in magazines as it is via broadcast outlets such as television and radio. Knowing this should shape your preparations for an interview in terms of what themes you think they will be interested in covering (whether facelifts or body contouring), but should NOT, in any shape or form alter your way of speaking or the colloquialisms you use. We will explore interview techniques soon.

Demographics are a key element to consider in proactive PR, particularly, when securing case studies. Case studies are, to put it simply, essential. The public are not going to just 'take your word for it' that this is the ideal treatment for 40-year-old women. Keep in mind who your target market is—is it men? How old are they? Is it baby boomers? Select case studies accordingly, aimed at the appropriate readership. Know that a 70-year-old man will never grace the cover of *GQ*. Know that a woman of indeterminate age, with mediocre before and afters, will never make it into *Marie Claire*. There is no point in yelling at your publicist about this.

CONSUMER HEALTH

In essence, you mostly have a captive audience in *some* of the health consumer publications and broadcast (TV and radio) outlets. They are probably already covering self-improvement and anti-aging. Some, however, may be anti-cosmetic surgery. I cannot reiterate it enough: KNOW YOUR AUDIENCE. Some outlets are very friendly towards aesthetic treatments (some really can't get enough), and others bemoan the fact that cosmetic surgery 'messes with nature'. Normally, I don't even approach these outlets, there is no point. Similarly, certain august broadsheets will always consider cosmetic surgery 'beneath them' and are unlikely to cover your offering.

But overall, magazines and TV/radio programmes dedicated to health and well-being will for the most part be receptive to your offering as long as it fits in with their audience. Get to know them—have a flick through the magazines at the airport or the supermarket. No one says you have to subscribe to *Company* (unless you happen to be, or feel like a 22-year-old woman and don't we all sometimes?) but it's worth knowing who you're speaking to. Whether you personally prefer the *Post* to the *Times*, be aware that there are specific sections and supplements that could be of relevance to you, for example in the U.K., the *Daily Mail* has regular sections such as 'Doctor Heal Thyself' or 'Me and My Operation' which are ideal showcases for your work and views. There are local and cable channels specifically tailored towards health and beauty subjects. The audience doesn't compare to *Oprah?* Well yes, but people watching or listening to a cosmetic surgery talk show will already be interested in cosmetic surgery to begin with!

OTHER SPECIALIST MAGAZINES

There's a plethora of publications out there that can present opportunities for you, if you can pinpoint stories that are of interest to them. Wedding magazines publish all year round—are there are treatments or case studies that are ideal for this market, that you could offer them? Are there any particular ethnic groups—Asian or Latina women—that are experiencing any interesting trends that you could highlight? What about the gay community? Parenting magazines? Business directors and entrepreneurs? What about general practitioners? There will be plenty of outlets aimed at all of these markets. Do you run marathons yourself, and is there a story to be weaved around this? Consider running or triathlon titles. If there's an international or cross-state market for you, consider, for example, the great number of airline and hotel magazines available. Always keep in mind, however, the mantra that they are not there to service *you*—so consider very carefully what material you can offer them that will knock their readers' socks off. Why would they write about you instead of one of their many advertisers? Make it worth their while—give 'em something juicy.

BLOGS

It would be absurd to ignore the growing permeation of bloggers and their vast influence. Nowadays information can be made so immediate, that certain high-profile writers of blogs (i.e., Web logs) are treated with as much if not more respect than mainstream journalists. There are, however, millions of people writing their own 'blogs'—including mainstream journalists themselves—and they see this medium as a way of bypassing traditional means and going straight to the public: unfiltered. But unfiltered also means that there is no vetting involved, no editors, which means that anyone can pretty much set up and run their own blog. Cosmetic surgery and aesthetic treatments can be a source of infinite interest to many of them, and they may well ask to 'try out' certain procedures for review. Just like we always say to patients, it is essential that you do your research! Check how many visitors their blog really has, how popular it is, to see whether it's worth giving someone a discount of hundreds or thousands of dollars in exchange for coverage (check Peer Index listings for a measure of their online authority). It may not always be of enough benefit to you so discuss pros and cons with your publicist and if you don't have one, feel free to ask the blogger directly for their own 'media kit'.

> *Idea: Have you thought of writing your own blog?*

CREATING A MEDIA LIST

By now you should have a more defined idea of the type of outlets you want to be targeting. For my clients, we always establish a 'wish list'—it doesn't mean we won't target any media outside that list, but these will be the ones where they wish to appear in the most and where our efforts will be focused.

Usually this list will encompass the top daily and Sunday newspapers, the highest-circulation regional outlets, the most popular women and men's lifestyle magazines, any particular websites, blogs or other publications specific to their target market (say, 40-year-old men or women over 50) and broadcast options such as TV chat shows.

Be realistic! There is no point having a hundred outlets listed, you won't be able to pitch each and every one of them with enough focus. Make sure you're selective for your 'wish list'—have second- and third-tier categories. The mix of media outlets will also change with every announcement, depending on who you're aiming for.

8 Tools of the trade

What channels are available to speak with the media? How—and when—do journalists expect to hear from you? This chapter will provide some handy rules for straightforward communication with journalists. It will give a comprehensive 'how-to' guide to creating a media kit and writing announcements, as well as alternative options such as holding a briefing on site.

PRESS KIT

Before launching any kind of PR campaign, one of the first things that you will need to put together is a press kit for you, your private practice or hospital. Back in the wild days of my youth, these revered and extensive packages generally took the form of hard copy pocket folders that contained press releases, previous cover- age, fact sheets and bios (all on real paper!). These were posted regularly to journalists, sometimes including branded promos such as beanie babies and mousemats (showing my age here). In fact, PR agencies would always try and come up with innovative ways for their materials to 'stick out' from the tons of press kits journalists would receive on a daily basis. I remember hearing of press releases 'written' on cookies and pizza! Certainly ensures that they will be looked at ...

The advantage of hard copies was that they would file these under a particular heading, and if/when the reporters were asked to write about, say, cosmetic dentistry or Botox, they would go and retrieve this information and look you up.

However, in these instant-response days of Google, MSN and WhatsApp, no one has time for snail mail. But the importance of having a comprehensive press kit remains—only now all the information should also be collated electronically and made easily available. Here is a generic list of 'start-up materials' ideal for anyone about to launch a PR campaign:

- Business Profile of the organisation and its history
- Executive Bios and photos of all spokespeople
- Fact Sheets (if relevant): listing of all products, treatments and services
- Previous press releases (announcements, partnerships, launches), if any
- Photography for stock library: high resolution photos of any equipment that will be promoted, facilities
- Personnel/staff photos, action shots if available—that is, the team performing procedures, meeting with patients and so on
- Case studies and before-and-after photos of treatments: Essential! (see 'Case Study' section in chapter 6)
- Existing relationships that may be leveraged: memberships, trade associations, links with recognised names or endorsements, celebrity connections, awards, etc.
- Time frame for announcements: will you be participating in any trade or consumer events? Are there any new products or treatments about to launch, or any new members joining your team? Are you moving facilities any time soon? Make sure you structure a timeline and plan accordingly (keep in mind media lead times!)
- Strategic Partners
- Marketing collateral: information brochures, print media
- Advertising (if any has taken place)
- Research: market assessment studies, industry analysis, relevant health and beauty statistics (percentage of people that suffer from the conditions you treat and so on)

To launch a publicity campaign without having all this information secured and at your fingertips is pretty risky. After you give them an idea for a story, journalists do not have time to wait while you dig out some old files and trawl through folders of Polaroids—by the time you locate the material they may have moved on. Or worse, used your story quoting a rival expert or their case study!

PRESS RELEASES

The way that we communicate with the press is, for the most part, through the humble medium of the press release. Of course, we also ring journalists and have long, rambling chats on the phone where we can wax lyrical on the merits of this or that treatment or expert … who am I kidding? They do not have time for that, *especially* newspaper journalists. So as publicists we have come to rely on this type of communication and I do not understate the matter when I say that some PRs have managed to elevate and hone this form to a sublime art. Good publicists worry obsessively about the placement of commas and the right synonym. Left unchecked, my team and I can debate headlines and the merit of puns for hours. Yes, we are nerds, in our own way …

One of the nicest compliments I've received in my career was from the medical editor of the *Sunday Times*, who said to me: "I can always tell when a press release comes from you, because everything I need to know is in the first paragraph." I nearly wept with pride because that, to be honest, is what a press release should do. It's down to the age-old journalism rules of Who, What, Where, When and Why.

So first off, we decided we had some news—there is something that needs to be shouted from the rooftops. We've outlined in a previous chapter what this type of news should (and shouldn't be). Whether it's a launch, or a partnership, or a safety warning, your headline, subheader and opening paragraph need to be an irresistible siren song. Journalists will be receiving thousands of press releases, and yours needs to somehow tower head and shoulders above the rest.

A fairly straightforward format that I tend to follow (and that's so far worked successfully for me) will always include the following elements, more or less in this specific order depending on the story:

- For Immediate Release (or embargo date)
- HEADLINE and Subheader
- First paragraph: Place–Date–Who, what (i.e., everything they need to know)

- Second paragraph: Further info (why)
- Third and Fourth: Expert/spokespeople comment
- Fifth: Conclusion, boilerplate

I try to keep press releases to a page, or a page-and-a-half at most.

For Immediate Release: Is the information free and available right now to publish? Or is there an 'embargo', in which case you need to clearly establish when exactly the information can be published. Embargoes are usually respected, but there is always the risk they could be broken. Personally, I try to go 'behind the scenes' and secure an exclusive first (which will pretty much guarantee you the exposure) then issue the release simultaneous to the coverage appearing, to give other media outlets the chance to subsequently run the story.

The objective here is to ensure that the press release has, literally, everything the journalist needs to write/present the story. Of course, you want them to interview you and thus be able to experience first-hand your many virtues and awe-inspiring knowledge, but I refer again to my previous point: they don't always have the time. When a press release is concise and well written, you have made the journalist's life easier. Once again, you are making them look good in front of their boss, editor or producer.

Just keep in mind that your press release is not meant to be written for the public—but for journalists. Having said that, journalists will also appreciate laymen terms and, when appropriate, a sense of humour!

Let's spend a little time on the headlines, because they are the first thing the journalist sees and they have to 'suck them in'. In the U.K., there is a higher preference for word-play than there is in the U.S., but regardless of puns, humour or alliteration being used (more on this later), it should give an indication of what's inside the tin. Here are some examples of headlines that are both eye catching and easy to grasp:

EXAMPLES

Warnings

SURGERY ONLINE COUPONS SLAMMED
Time-linked incentives violate code of ethics, say surgeons

BEWARE THE NUT JOB
Warning over Unlicensed Male Genital Enhancement

Statistics

BRITONS OVER THE MOOB
Male Breast Reduction Figures Nearly Double

THIS IS A MAN'S WORLD: MOOBS AND THE DREADED
COMBOVER
Survey of men's aesthetic worries

New procedures

FOR YOUR ABS ONLY: GET A BODY LIKE BOND
Body sculpting technique gives carved, muscled look the easy way

BACK ROLLS AND MUFFIN TOPS
Latest liposuction techniques for those hard-to-reach places

New products

COOL RUNNINGS
Post-Surgery Cooling Therapy Delivered to Your Door

MEDICAL APP-OINTMENTS ON THE MOVE
*New Health care App Allows You to Search, Compare and Book
Private Treatment*

I think you probably get the idea of what each story will cover just
by reading the headline. The point is to convince journalists that

what you're about to tell them, will make their bosses happy and help sell magazines. It's a fairly straightforward premise but can take time to perfect. If you can make the journalist intrigued—or even make them laugh (for the right reasons) while they're at it, even better.

Opening paragraphs

The first paragraph should have everything they need to know. First of all, you need to state clearly WHEN and WHERE you're issuing this announcement from. Is it coming from London or New York? Birmingham (Alabama or U.K.)? Perth (Scotland or Australia)? As well as the date. Before your opening sentence, establish:

Boston, Massachusetts—June 6th, 2012

Tunbridge Wells, Kent—April 4th, 2011

And so on. Then launch into your most concise and pithy first paragraph. Enough should be in the opener that journalists can instantly tell whether it's relevant to them. Don't wait until the third or fourth paragraph because they might not make it that far ...

EXAMPLES

A private clinic of over 60 leading psychiatrists, psychologists and psychotherapists, today unveil the results of an online survey that polled women who have, or have had, the controversial PIP implants. It revealed that well over half of women had missed work due to stress over having PIPs, nearly 8 out of 10 feel their self-esteem and self-worth have been affected, two-thirds are feeling severely depressed and anxious and 80% feel they will need the help of a therapist of counsellor. Nearly all (92%) are suffering from insomnia.

Women suffering a protruding 'mummy tummy' following pregnancy and birth may have more to worry about than just a little extra baby weight. According to a leading plastic surgeon, between

10% and 15% of women suffer a hernia during pregnancy, which they are often unaware of. If left undetected and untreated, the problem can worsen and can even result in weakening and eventual rupturing of the stomach wall.

Excessive sweating can be a problem all year round, but particularly insufferable in the summer. While many of us can curb underarm sweating with a good anti-perspirant, sufferers of Hyperhidrosis are plagued with the problem continually—which often cannot be solved with deodorants and may force them to shower many times throughout the day, greatly affecting their lives and confidence. A leading cosmetic doctor highlights the little-known use of Botox to cure the condition—a tried and tested method which has changed the lives of many, including 32-year-old local resident X.

QUOTES

Why is it important to have quotes in a press release? Why not simply present the information to them like an essay or academic paper? Once again, it is all about making the journalist's life easier. The quicker they can cobble your story together and the less research they have to conduct on their own, the better. Of course, in an ideal world they will spend a long time on the phone with you, to get extra insight into the themes being highlighted—but the best scenario is to give them a pre-packaged story that has all the elements they will need, should they not have time to speak with you in detail. Make sure you always fully identify the expert speaking with their correct title and relevant information such as membership to organisations that will add credibility: for example, 'According to Dr. X, a [board-certified] [dermatologist/surgeon], member of the American/British Relevant Organisation]', similarly with the case studies: 'According to Y, a 32-year-old secretary who resides in Z'.

EXAMPLES

> *"The procedure isn't suitable for everyone, such as those with poor skin tone, but we are always happy to advise patients on the best treatment options for them, to*

ensure they get the best results possible. No one should be able to guess that you've had surgery—they'll think you've just worked out."

"The number of women who would consider surgery abroad is certainly worrying. We firmly believe cosmetic surgery should be carried out by a well researched, reputable surgeon as, even in the best hands, surgery can be challenging and complicated. Aftercare is paramount and patients should find out as much information as possible about their surgeon. Once the patient returns home from surgery abroad aftercare is limited and any problems are difficult and costly to overcome. If complications occur patients can at best find themselves paying more than if they'd had the surgery at home and at worst have a terrible result which compromises their health."

"I was aware of the problems with PIPs for much longer than a lot of women who didn't find out until last December—I had been following the reports in the media and discovered I had these implants back in June 2010. Over time I became increasingly anxious and frustrated with the situation and the clinic I had undergone the operation with who were doing nothing to help women like myself. Although eventually (under Government pressure) they have ended up offering a 'rescue' deal for half the usual amount, at the time that wasn't the case. I would have had to find the full cost of £5000 for PIP replacement surgery which I simply did not have."

"When someone loses a lot of weight like this patient has, excess skin is inevitable as it has stretched so much and loses elasticity. The only option in these cases is surgery. Sometimes an abdominoplasty (tummy tuck) is enough but since a tummy tuck involves a hip to hip incision, any excess tissues further round are not excised and can result in looking like 'dog ears' at each hip. In these cases only a body lift will restore shape. The body lift involves cutting all the way around the body, removing the excess tissue and re-attaching it to the trunk."

"I'm fairly active and eat healthily but I've never been able to shift these stubborn pockets of fat, no matter what I do. I would never have considered liposuction under a general anaesthetic and with a hospital stay, but when I heard about the XYZ Laser*

*treatment it sounded ideal. Being able to have a local anaes-
thetic and undergo the procedure in a clinic environment with
no hospital stay appealed to me—and the reduced downtime
was a real bonus. I didn't even have sedation and the procedure went fine and I was up and about straight afterwards.
I was slightly sore but nothing worse than what you'd feel after
a good gym workout and the next day I was out walking the dog
as usual. I'm delighted with the results."*

Boilerplates

Remember that the body of your press release should have everything they need. At the end of the release, you will want to add a
short 'boilerplate', which doesn't tend to have a formal structure
but is just a short paragraph about you. It is simply for the refer-
ence of the editors, a little overview of the organisation or the clinician involved in the story. What services are provided, address
and phone number for appointments, and who journalists should
contact in case of any queries. If you have a PR agent, their details
should be included here, to avoid your clinical staff fielding time-
consuming enquiries from the media.

> *Tip: Don't use obscure acronyms in your press releases, and
> always explain any medical terminology.*

MEDIA BRIEFINGS

A lot of clients want to hold press events. They feel—nay, they
know—that should the journalist be exposed directly to the sun-
beam of their charm they will not be able to resist writing article
after article about their talent and expertise. Some even still hold
to the antiquated adage of 'have booze and they will come', and
whilst this holds true for college kids (well OK, and maybe me),
this is no longer the case with serious journalists. Even the most
groundbreaking media briefings, with announcements that have
repercussions far and wide, have to justify any time spent away
from their desk. In these increasingly straitened times, they have
to convince their bosses that they need to be in situ when the
news breaks. Time is money for everyone.

In certain instances, it is inarguable that the best thing you can do is invite the media to meet with you face to face. But it has to be something worth their while—we'll examine here various options as to why and when it might be more advantageous to have the media come to you at a designated venue, rather than just receiving press releases and information by email. The encounter can take place at your office or hospital, during a trade show (perhaps a demonstration at your booth if you're launching a new product) or at a formal events venue where you can hold a press conference.

I do struggle sometimes when clients feel that the press will clearly come in droves to examine their jazzy new premises or coo at new non-surgical lipo machine. Really ask yourself if you're giving them something of value (or refer to 'p*ssing down your own leg' section).

The main, overriding reason why you would invite journalists to discuss some new development for a media briefing or a 'press day', is because they need to be able to ask you questions directly, face-to-face. Perhaps the information is quite extensive, or the science quite involved, and journalists would benefit from being in a room with you to explain it. I've had to hold press conferences about a series of complex operations taking place on a high-profile case, and the media needed diagrams and direct access to the specialists involved. Setting up a press conference for something so groundbreaking can take months of preparation, with slides and models and extensive negotiations as to who gets access to what. In this instance, I got to witness some very respectable journalists fighting like snarling dogs over photos and film footage! My therapist feels it best if I don't focus on that particular period of my life, but just know that press days aren't always something that you can throw together at the last minute.

The main societies for aesthetic plastic surgery and for cosmetic medicine hold annual meetings and generally have at least one open 'Press Day', where journalists are invited to attend and learn about the latest developments in the profession. In some, the media are even invited to attend the scientific sessions but this is not always the case, due to patient confidentiality issues.

However, the great majority do hold a general briefing where they can provide an overview of the themes that are being covered. The importance of maintaining this type of open-door policy cannot be underestimated, even if it does make some clinicians grumble. Access helps journalists keep abreast of the latest news, but more importantly you thus earn their goodwill; it shows a willingness to share advances with the public that has an endless fascination with all things cosmetic, and makes reporters feel adequately informed. No one likes feeling like they came late to a party. Developing a relationship in which you gain their trust is invaluable.

It's worth noting that having members of the press come to you doesn't automatically guarantee you an easy ride. First off, they have to justify the time and effort it took to be present, and don't want to go back to their desks admitting they entirely misjudged the matter and their day was a waste. They will have questions that will need an answer publicly, without the shelter of email, and occasionally depending on what outlet they work for they may even be outright hostile. But the gesture of allowing them in is, in itself, a show of goodwill and openness. Let's not kid ourselves, many a scathing article has been written poking fun at conferences full of slick-looking doctors and trout-pouted exhibitors, but it has to be accepted that they will be writing about the sector anyways—potentially even sneaking in if not invited! (it's happened)—so you may as well extend the olive branch.

A different level of media briefing is where a clinic or company wants to showcase a new product, skincare range or machine. If you are exhibiting at a trade show or speaking at a conference, it is likely that journalists will be attending anyways, and it's up to you to capitalise on this footfall. Find out from the organisers which day is 'Press Day', and whether you can schedule demonstrations. Have your publicist contact members of the press that might be likely to attend, and invite them to meet with you at a designated time for a chat. Usually there will be a designated room where you can leave literature, samples and press kits for the media. Some of the most famous skincare brands, for example, tend to leave goody bags at events. One year at a client's Annual Conference, the Press Room descended into something vaguely resembling the IKEA riots, with journalists fighting over freebies. Ah, spare a thought for the health care journalist. As one medical editor put it to me: "I never get good stuff from PRs—last week I was sent an STD home-testing kit …."

Follow up!

Every point of contact is an opportunity. If you chatted with a journalist at an event, make sure you take their contact details and stay in touch with them. They receive so many press kits and news releases that they're likely to forget (though I'm sure of course you're very memorable). In the next chapter we'll examine how to 'pitch' stories to them.

Another option to personally brief the media is to invite them to your premises, perhaps to undergo a treatment themselves or witness one being performed. However, always check that what you're offering is of value TO THEM. Not just to you and your business. Are you giving them an amazing story that will knock their editors' socks off? One of the editors of a major Sunday newspaper once said to me: "I want stories that people will talk about later at the pub."

So, the main question to ask yourself is, can the same information and news be sent via email and phone? The answer shouldn't be what you'd prefer—what is most convenient to you—but (here's a thought) what would actually be the most convenient to them.

Consider the journalists' time to be as valuable as your own.

In the past I was outbid for a client contract by an agency that promised lots and lots of 'bums on seats' for a launch event. I've always been honest and said "I concentrate on results and achieving coverage," but won't focus all my efforts in just getting random people to attend. As much as it may please your vanity to look out upon a packed room of media representatives listening to you, make sure they're not just there for the free canapés and that those pens aren't just doodling. Personally, I have found no direct correlation between quorum and the coverage that ensues. This is why so many organisations, including this client —who eventually came back to us—can be disappointed after they invest the time and money to hold a big flashy briefing. These events can be well attended (especially if it's at an elegant venue and there's champagne involved), but may still result in tumbleweed on the media front. Always consider the effort versus possible return.

Obviously I am not saying don't hold a press day if you want to meet and greet the media, but be open to other options depending on the strength of the announcement you have to make. Would it make more sense to stagger the open days, so that journalists can come at *their* convenience? As always, keep in mind that just because they came, it doesn't necessarily mean they'll feature you. This is when a publicist really comes into their own, and they can pursue leads, ensure that the right information has been received, and generally make a pest of themselves (we're good at that sort of thing, it's a gift).

9 Pitching to journalists

By now you've hopefully pinpointed something newsworthy to say, and a particular group of people who should know about it. How to approach a journalist and convince them that their audience will find it of interest?

It's rather unlikely that you as clinicians will find yourselves making the first call to pitch a story directly to a journalist. This will be the job of your PR—if you have one—or perhaps your Marketing person or even your Practice Manager. Nevertheless, it's important that you understand what's involved and how the process of selling a story works, so that not only you don't find yourself stumped down the line (why won't they write about me?) but also realise how it works from their end. Knowing how to sell a premise to a journalist can always come in handy, as you might find yourself casually in conversation with them either at a social function or perhaps answering a 'reactive' request. You can then use some tricks of the trade to *ninja* them with another angle while you're at it.

As in any environment, there is an established hierarchy in journalism, from researchers to assistants, reporters, producers and editors. There are news, health, features and beauty beats. There are dedicated sections and columns, and it's not always easy to determine who might be the ideal contact to pitch to. When I am given some material by a client, I can usually, by instinct, know what outlets might be interested. But is it news or is it health? Is it the Women's section or is it Science?

Publicists will have access to enormous databases of media contacts—these are either honed over time or paid-for subscription services. Most agencies will have developed a combination of both, which is why I stress the importance of selecting an agency that specialises in your sector. There is no point in hiring publicists that know everyone in fashion, or food and drink, or hospitality. Personally, I have direct access to well over a thousand close, trusted journalist contacts that I have worked with over the last decade, and I keep careful records of who has covered what stories. But there are also companies that sell lists that automatically update themselves as editors and reporters move around—which they undoubtedly do and very regularly.

It may seem counterintuitive, if you're first wading into the murky waters of PR, to start with lower strata of hierarchy, like health or feature assistants. But more often than not, the way it works in media is that journalists as a team sit in planning meetings (whether it's newspapers, magazines or TV or radio programmes) to discuss what ideas can be featured or might be of interest. Everyone is generally expected to bring suggestions to the table. Making a lowly assistant look good by offering them a unique opportunity to pitch to their bosses will earn their long-time gratitude. I have lost count of the amount of times that I've discovered this or that correspondent at a regional paper eventually becomes a hot-shot Editor or Producer with a high-profile outlet. These are contacts I have made for life, and I've become close friends with many of them over time. I remember meeting a young correspondent from a local newspaper who attended the first media briefing I ever organised. We fell into conversation and stayed in touch. The next few years she continued to attend our conferences, and always impressed with extensive articles about the advances in cosmetic surgery. She was eventually made the Health Editor of that particular regional newspaper, and soon after, it was announced that she'd take over as Medical Editor for one of the most prestigious broadsheets in the U.K. We are still good friends, and we've developed enough trust in each other that I can speak 'off-the-record' and brainstorm ideas with her. Another freelancer who used to write features for Scottish news agency was eventually made the Commissioning Editor of one of the most popular women's magazines. Social media such as Twitter has also connected me with fantastic journalists around the globe, from South Africa to California, New York and Australia.

There are plenty of free websites where you can look up media contact details, and many newspapers and outlets will actually list their editorial teams. In magazines, you can always flick thru the pages to the masthead, which will list the editorial staff.

> Bad pick-up lines: *You know what would look great in your paper? Me.*

WHO TO SPEAK WITH?

When it's REACTIVE, there will be a journalist at the other end of the phone or email, who is the health/medical writer, a features or even news editor. They are already working on a piece, so help them get this out of the way first. Feel free to ask what other kinds of pieces they write, and suggest you may have other similar stories that their audience (i.e., their boss) might be interested in. In this instance the process is fairly straightforward, talk to the person that's writing the article.

When it's PROACTIVE, it's a bigger decision and it can be easy to get bogged down trying to pinpoint the right contact, who is working on the right story, at the right time. The reason why good publicists secure a lot of coverage is because they are constantly in touch with the media. They know who is working on what— they speak with Commissioning Editors regularly and know the sort of thing magazines are after. Personally, I can look at a story and instantly know which outlet or journalist would find it of relevance.

So at the top of the food chain of course we have editors, who are usually very busy and have minions they can delegate to. Writers and correspondents will be frantically scrabbling at good, solid stories that will help them keep their viewer numbers or readership and circulation up. There are also armies of freelancers—many who specialise in specific types of outlets such as women's magazines or Sunday newspapers.

Initially you might think—OK I've followed the magical PR sequence: I've got a good story, written up in a concise press release, and I know which magazine/newspaper/TV show I want to appear in. Feel free to contact the general switchboard and ask "who covers health?" or, "who would be the best person to talk to about a local clinic's charity fundraising?" etc. The issue is that, sometimes, there is often more than one contact that can be appropriate.

Just because Health doesn't want to cover it, Features might. Or News. So it can be a bit of a guessing game and certainly involves a lot of trial and error. This, again, is why experienced publicists are invaluable. In particular, publicists who are known for one particular sector such as cosmetic surgery. They will know that sometimes the Business reporter will be covering news from this arena, sometimes it will be Home Affairs or even Culture & Society. These are all separate beats and each journalist jealously guards what is given to them. Consider the list of angles—is there a Technology or Science editor? A 'Woman' section?

How to p*ss them off

One theme which has proven recurrent among many journalists is outright revulsion towards experts who complain about *other* experts they might choose to quote in their articles. "If there are safety concerns about a product I'm plugging, or you know there's a genuine problem with a clinic, then I'm open to feedback," a top freelancer who writes for national Sunday newspapers said to me. "But to just whinge about a 'rival' being featured will ensure that I never use you again."

I have asked in the past high-profile journalists who regularly write about cosmetic surgery what would categorically ensure that they NEVER cover a certain doctor, surgeon, procedure or clinic.

"Arrogance," one said, rolling her eyes. "I know you're great, but let's be frank, you're not saving the world one nose job at a time."

Another issue cited by journalists when I asked about their turn-offs was "implausible" or "murky" scientific data. Matt Barbour, a contributing editor to U.K. tabloid *The Sun* (and the 10th highest circulation newspaper in the world), explains what would turn him off:

"No specifics on a 'story' (new procedure, etc.) explaining how it's new, why it's better than the conventional treatment. For a clinic or doctor I need to know their specific areas of expertise, and direct contact information so I know I can get in touch when needed."

And what he's after:

"I would look for fully identified case studies and strong data backing up claims. My editors expect to the point, pithy pitches highlighting the benefits to the reader, with case studies of the right demographic for the publication."

A conversation with top cosmetic surgery reporter and freelancer Leah Hardy, an ex-editor of *Cosmopolitan* magazine, who regularly writes for many national newspapers such as the *Mail on Sunday*, the *Guardian* and glossy magazines such as *Red, Easy Living* and *Grazia*:

"What would guarantee that you never look at a treatment, clinic or doctor?"

Big red flags for me are if I heard bad word of mouth about lack of aftercare, shoddy or callous treatment or if they were more concerned with pushing a product from a company rather than the actual interests of their patients. Other problems for me are people who have had bad or excessive work on their own faces—that would put me off! In particular those who complain about their coverage for stupid reasons, such as the feature also featured 'rival' doctors or surgeons.

"What do you look for in a press release from them?"

The absolutely ideal, could-place-it-yesterday press release gives me a new product, technique or a new use for an existing product. It tells me why it is superior to previous treatments, tells me that a celebrity has used or endorsed it, there is a link to something topical in the news (e.g., the Pippa bottom!) and you have an attractive, aspirational case study already lined up.

"What would convince you to write about them?"

See above! Also, I have to admit, I have doctors, surgeons and PRs that I trust. It's a lot of put your face in the hands of someone you don't know. It would help to tell me qualifications, professional memberships, and link me to scientific papers about the studies, treatments or product.

"What are some of the best pitches you've ever had?"

One of the best pitches involved a new liposuction technique to create a Pilates body inspired by Pippa Middleton—I could practically guarantee a front-page splash. Sadly it didn't work out because at the last minute the patient pulled out. Being offered an exclusive—and it really, genuinely being an exclusive—very much helps. I'll work harder to place it. I have to say, most of my features are based on my own ideas and angles, but of course I also rely on information gathered from PR sources. Worst pitches? I'd say anything too dull …

"What are your editors and readers expecting from you?"

My editors expect something new—which can be difficult as we all know that the newer the treatment, the less tried it is and so the risks are greater for the public. Alternatively they also look for a topical angle, so a new study from overseas or a celebrity trend could work well as the hook, but the celebs do need to be current and famous. Editors often love anything with a shock-horror angle too. So if your treatment sounds a bit gruesome (e.g., Dracula Therapy) they will love it. Cautionary tales such as treatments going wrong are always appealing to editors, if not necessarily to doctors! My readers want to know about solutions to their everyday problems or challenges, they want to obtain recommendations for doctors and treatments that are effective and safe. As you can see, all these demands can be hard to reconcile.

One of the most common complaints about cosmetic surgery reporting is that a lot of it is greatly sensationalised, with little grasp of the science behind procedures. Less-savvy journalists can be easily impressed or swayed by exaggerated claims. But with recent developments such as the PIP saga in Europe and Latin America, and a number of cosmetic injectables being taken off the market, there is hopefully a growing culture of healthier scepticism, which can only be a good thing for the public in the long run.

As legendary U.S. journalist Joan Kron (of *Allure* magazine's famous 'Scalpel News') once said to me "Every time I mention a doctor, I know I'm putting someone on their operating table." Some journalists clearly take their responsibilities more seriously than others.

In PR, as in life, flattery will almost always help. If you have time before an interview or before approaching a journalist for the first time, look up what else they have covered in the past. You will seem much more clued up if you say "I enjoyed the piece you did last month on nose teeth whitening/swine flu/bunions." They will be pleasantly surprised.

When pitching a story, it's also important to understand how the media environment works and under what pressures they operate. It's unusual to find a newspaper journalist, for example, willing to have a long chat late in the afternoon. They're almost always going to be on deadline for the next day's paper. Sunday newspapers and magazines—anything with a longer lead—will have more time. Either way, most of them will appreciate information sent by email, with a follow-up call a day or two later. They will not appreciate a call five minutes after to check if they received it!

Having said that—it is of course important to respect their schedules—be persistent. Journalists are busy people and newsrooms can get quite frantic. The thing about PR is that it will be affected by what's happening elsewhere. If there is a series of explosive world events, there will be less column inches to spare for health and fuzzy features. And if there's a huge development in another area of medicine (say, in diabetes, in vitro fertilisation or heart disease), well you may as well wave goodbye to your hand rejuvenation story for the time being. At the height of the PIP crisis, when a lack of regulation is highlighted and injectables are being pulled off the market or banned, it is no wonder that your feel-good story about the difference wrinkle smoothing has made to someone's life and forehead doesn't make it into *Time* magazine.

There are, and have been, controversial stories that make front-page splashes. I have secured more of these in my career that I can recall off the top of my head. Themes that really catch the audience's attention and, in the editor's immortal words "stuff they'll talk about at the pub" will never fail to secure a good spread. I've made the entire front page of Sunday newspapers with a study about the addictive traits of Botox users (a paper presented at a surgery conference), as well as the reaction from surgeons that cosmetic surgery was to be taxed (known in the U.S. as Bo-Tax).

So by all means find the best contact and send your press release. Give them a few days then call up to ensure they received it. Offer interviews and photos. A tip: do NOT send big attachments unsolicited. They will only clog up their inbox and annoy them. Also, really question the use of images that you may include in your press releases. The illustration or diagram of a theory posited in the release makes sense—a close-up photo of Michelangelo's David's penis will only cause much hilarity (and circulated as a joke to other PRs).

Be persistent, however. Don't trust them to remember who you are—perhaps they won't be writing about cosmetic surgery this month, but they may well be next.

STAFF VERSUS FREELANCERS

The main difference is self-explanatory—staff will be paid whether they place a story or not, and freelancers will ONLY get paid if they place a story. There are pros and cons to using each. The freelancers may well be more motivated, because they know that if they manage to convince an editor to run their article, it's pay day for them. A slight disadvantage is that once it's handed over to the editors, they won't be able to tell you necessarily when it will be used. Staff, on the other hand, will have more control over the process and will know where the piece might be in the 'queue'. Depending on the story, I always think of the ideal freelancer or staff editor who would be most appropriate.

DIY PR: PRACTISE AT HOME!

There was an exercise that my old boss used to make us practice, when I worked at a PR agency in New York City (man, them were the days … big budgets, Swarovski jewellery sent out in press kits … OK I may be exaggerating a little). This involved taking an imaginary business or brand, and pitching it to different outlets that would clearly require different angles. It's actually a great way of exploring how you can promote your own offering to different media at the same time.

For the purposes of this industry, let's pick a fairly standard and popular procedure, like for example, treatment for acne. Let's say we have a magnificent new STAR WARS laser. What do you suppose you need to tell the following outlets, to convince them to write about this? Think carefully about the product attributes that you would trot out to each of these:

- Cosmopolitan
- Financial Times
- OK!
- Men's Health

- Good Housekeeping
- Reader's Digest
- The Liverpool Daily Echo

Stuff to think about: are there high-profile name endorsements that could help the treatment seem attractive to a gossip magazine? Are bankers and stockbrokers 'breaking out' more because of stress and the recession? Is there a rise in acne among men or those who practice sport? Do over 50s get acne? Be as creative as you like!

> *Always consider—who would be the most appropriate case study for these outlets?*

Now apply the same to a dermal lip filler or new liposuction technique. How can you make the former appeal to your local newspaper, or the latter be of interest to a high-fashion male magazine such as GQ?

> *Put yourself in the journalists' shoes—what would they want to know? What will make them a good story?*

EXCLUSIVES

You needn't be a brain surgeon to figure this one out; it basically means you offer it to one person first. Offering journalists a story can be a complex balance game with a bit of cat-and-mouse flirting thrown in. Most journalists will turn their nose up at a press release that's been carpet-bombed to 900 contacts. They'll think, "Hey, I'm not special. Everyone has this press release. I won't bother." Yet, to individually contact each prospect, and wait until they run it past their editors, then get back to you with feedback (which could well be a 'maybe') can be extremely time-consuming. However, it invariably yields the best results. A newspaper or TV programme that feels they have a head start over anyone else, will be perceived as 'clued-up' and therefore earn your gratitude.

One thing that will instantly discredit you as unprofessional or an amateur is—whether intentionally or not—pitting two or more journalists against each other for the same story. Not only will you enrage them (and probably ensure they never, ever write up any of your stories), but you may also infuriate the editor that's at the receiving end of various freelancers offering the same piece. It is bad form. Make sure that a journalist has turned down your story (or you've given them enough time to respond) *before* offering it to the next.

Remember that what happens in the news—even outside of health and beauty—will affect journalists' receptiveness (negatively or positively) towards your pitch. So, if your story happens to be tied in with something topical: the recession, the Royal Wedding, annual surgery statistics, the PIP implant saga, the elections or something seasonal (bikini bodies? Party season treatments? New Year, New You?) it will more likely be considered as a relevant, 'current' subject.

> *If tying your news release to something topical, make sure the 'link' is actually genuine!*

Getting a 'hit', that is, securing coverage, can be quite a serendipitous process. You may ring this editor today and they can categorically say that there is absolutely no interest in covering cosmetic surgery or aesthetic treatments at all. Next week this may change, and they probably won't backtrack and call you but simply use whoever is contacting them at the time. Also, outlets that historically haven't proven friendly to cosmetic surgery may undergo a change in direction and decide that, after all, it is something that they're interested in. This happens a lot when there's a new editor or producer in charge. It's a fluid environment and things are constantly changing, and space for a story can suddenly open up last minute, which is why good publicists are always on the move—it is rarely a 9-to-5 job!

PRESS RELEASE DISTRIBUTION SERVICES, NEWSWIRES AND SEARCH ENGINE OPTIMISATION

Many agencies these days can post your press release online via paid-for distribution services (such as Business Wire, MyNewsDesk, PRWeb), which will automatically make it available to thousands of websites and RSS feeds in one go. However, doing so before approaching mainstream journalists generally means that they will not pick this up! The main difference between these subscription wires and 'real' newswires such as Associated Press (AP), Reuters and Press Association (PA) (from which newspapers around the world get their news) is that the release doesn't undergo any editing, or really much vetting in any way before it's posted. To have a press release on PA, AP, etc.—or indeed newspapers like the *Wall Street Journal* and *The Guardian*—you have to 'sell' it to their journalists first, before posting it online for all and sundry.

This is why most PR agencies these days consider the unfiltered 'PR wires' or distribution services to be purely a Search Engine Optimisation (SEO) tool rather than a media relations one, regardless of having 'PR' in their name. You may get a lot of online coverage, which will 'bump' your Google rankings, but it will not necessarily help you achieve coverage in the most 'viral' news outlets. There are also unique requirements in terms of keywords to ensure that a press release helps with your SEO, which is why sometimes you'll find announcements on the Web seem to be very oddly written. This is the down to the expertise of your Web team, and pitching for SEO and pitching for mainstream media such as TV, newspapers and magazines are two very different areas.

SUMMARY

- Finding contact details for the media: look on the Web, browse the news stands
- Don't be shy and ask: Who is the best person to speak with?
- Walking the line between sections: medical, health, beauty, news, features, culture and society, Women's section, special supplements …
- Read up on what they've done in the past: "I enjoyed your article on …"
- Email and phone, but give time to review materials
- Stay focused—don't give up. If they don't hear from you after a while, they will not beat a path to your door
- Keep in mind their particular audience: pitching to *Hello!* Magazine is very different from pitching to the *Financial Times!!*
- Putting yourself in the journalist's shoes … what would they want to know?

10   Interview techniques

Now you have the journalist's attention (whether this is what you set out to do or not!). This section covers dealing directly with an interview situation and what is expected from you: the expert.

This is the point where a lot of people tend to panic—it's easy to fall into a 'they're out to get me/trip me up' tailspin. Let's remind ourselves what the journalist is after: knowledge, expertise, information, opinion, illumination, explanations …

Don't forget that *they* need *you*. They can't very well write a story along the lines of 'this is the best treatment for wrinkly foreheads/ it's dangerous to undergo buttock enlarging injections in someone's apartment … according to no one'. It is in their interest to get the best out of you, to secure good quotes that bring their item to life. As a top newspaper journalist said, when I asked why they always choose a specific surgeon for their interviews: "He gets it," she said simply. "He always gives me good, solid sound bites (more on this later), and most importantly, he picks up the phone."

Once you do well with a particular journalist, they will ask for your help time and again. Morning chat shows, as you can imagine, have their favourite 'resident experts' (more on this later as well). It becomes a near impossible task, in fact, to convince them to use anyone else, should that expert not be available for a specific opportunity, because they don't want to take risks. They know that someone who does well on camera, doesn't get flustered with difficult questions and is personable makes the viewers feel relaxed.

Regardless of their unique expertise (or having a face better suited to radio), their authority shines through. Help them make good TV!

We know who they are—as mentioned in chapter 2, the meteoric rise of the TV Doctor over the last decade is impossible to ignore. It is a testament to the sometimes desperate need of the public and media to have experts who can shed light on developments that sometimes we can be flummoxed even by the choice of expert. I have lost count of the amount of times clients have whined: "But he/she is a GP/Dermatologist/Nurse/vascular/ENT! What do they know about chemical peels/lasers/abdominoplasty/blepharo-plasty/stem cells??" The reality is, if that programme needs an 'expert' opinion, they will most likely use someone they've used before because they don't want to risk having someone boring or who comes across as nervous. They won't always ask probing questions about qualifications and training because they have a different set of objectives (although in the current climate this is improving). This could well be a failing on the part of the media—rage all you want—but

(a) remember they're there to sell a story, not to educate or inspire;
(b) the failing, if there is one, lies more on the lack of regulation that exists in the world of cosmetic surgery;
(c) never forget Clarke's 4th Law: for every expert, there is an equal and opposite expert!

I would like to be able to tell you that the media takes its vetting duties seriously every time, but journalists are human like you and I, and just as (or more) pressurised and rushed. They never signed up to a Hippocratic oath!

The bottom line is, you may be livid if what you consider to be an unsuitably qualified practitioner is offering a procedure you believe they're not trained to do but in the majority of cases, as it stands in most countries, they are breaking no laws. It puts publicists in a very difficult position sometimes, when we're told to pass on a complaint to TV producers about their choice of 'experts' if, technically, no one is doing anything illegal however unethical it might be considered. There is also a growing trend in cosmetic surgery 'advisors' or brokers that style themselves as experts and 'one of the people', as if not having gone to med school actually makes them better suited to advise the public. Whingeing about this to the media however, simply makes us look churlish.

> *It is your role to educate, inspire and promote safety. Not the media's. Feel strongly about something? Use the press strategically as a mouthpiece to reach thousands if not millions of people. Beat the cowboys at their own game!*

As publicists we have unofficial categories for our many spokespeople (that we would protect with our lives), and we know which experts do well in what type of media: Plain-Speaking Surgeon may be well suited to some opportunities, Suave TV Doctor and Housewives' Favourite for others. Sometimes the ones that get used time and again are chosen because they have a natural ability, with others it's a talent honed over years of being in the spotlight. I've had clients who were absolutely terrified of speaking with the press—and I mean breaking into a sweat and literally shaking—but after undergoing media training sessions they at least are able to get some practice under their belts and, if not enjoy the process, at least are able to get through it without too much anxiety. Not everyone likes being in the public eye. Some, clearly, relish the opportunity for whatever reason, because it helps their business or even just appeals to good old-fashioned vanity. Either way, there are techniques that can be learned to make media relations a relatively painless affair.

Some clinicians are anathema to smooth-talking media darlings and pride themselves on their candid—even blunt—approach. This can, in itself, be a strength. Plain-Speaking Surgeon's irascibility can be vaguely endearing and many journalists actually enjoy his no-nonsense pronouncements, but Politically Incorrect Doctor is best kept hidden, and we all have a Last Resort spokesperson (but hold onto your hats if we're reduced to those circumstances!).

What the message boils down to, once again, is that the media want a good story and to get the best from the interviewee. Except for very unusual circumstances, they just want to get some solid, concise quotes that will enhance their feature. It is in their interest to keep you on side, for the next time!

So to recap what we've covered previously, focus on what do journalists need:

- Knowledge
- Expertise
- Information
- Opinion
- Illumination
- Explanation

In short, they want:

- A good story
- To get the best from you

REMEMBER: They need you as much as you need them!

WHAT WILL THE JOURNALIST DO TO GET WHAT THEY WANT?

Friendly questions

Most of the time, they will have no reason to try anything but the friendly approach. It gets the best out of you, and involves less effort on their part. I've been making a big case here stressing that journalists aren't the enemy—but remember that doesn't mean they're your friend either! Acting like your best pal is a technique like any other, which they learn throughout their careers (some better than others). As long as you're giving them what they need, it's unlikely they will try any other, more 'underhanded' ways of getting information from you.

Aggressive questions

Depending on the outlet, the audience, and what they're covering, the journalist may well open quite aggressively instead. An outlet or audience that by principle is dead set against cosmetic surgery (feel that we're messing with nature, that people should grow old gracefully, that cosmetic doctors and surgeons are a bunch of body Nazis, whatever) might open the interview with full-on guns blazing. With the recent PIP implant scandal, I always had to be careful which spokespeople I sent where, because the opening gambit could easily be along the lines of "How could YOU (Surgeons/doctors/clinic owners) let this happen!?"

Depending on the debate taking place, you could well be a lamb delivered to the slaughter. Slightly like an overprotective mom, I sometimes worry about sending clients who are going to defend cosmetic surgery to certain audiences that I know will be attacking them. I always have to weigh the options—does it make us look better to engage with these groups and at least have a say?

A saying I've heard time and again, and which I subscribe to wholeheartedly is "the world is run by those who show up." So, stand up and be counted, I say. Participate. But maybe don't send Last Resort Guy.

As publicists we will usually know what to expect, and should brief you accordingly. Sometimes, journalists can *start* very friendly, so the interviewee feels relaxed, and then they become aggressive to catch them unawares. I cannot stress enough: always be on your guard. They are not there to trip you up, but don't let your tongue run away with you, either. I am continually shocked by what some professionals will let 'slip' when talking to a journalist. We will provide some tricks of the trade further on.

Repeated questions

A journalist who feels you are not giving a straight answer—or at least, you're not giving the answer they wish to hear—may choose to repeat the question, perhaps even more than once, worded each time in a slightly different way. The most famous example of this I can recall is when the BBC *Newsnight* presenter and famous journalist Jeremy Paxman asked his interviewee the same question FOURTEEN TIMES in a row. This was, of course, directed at a politician (who still remarkably managed to evade answering each time) so it is unlikely you will find yourself in this situation. But here we will explore ways of dealing with them.

Accusations

Journalists can be sneaky and this will come as no surprise. The weapons in their arsenal can be straightforward accusations that may or may not have any actual basis in fact. They may not even make any sense! If their objective is to get a rise out of you for whatever reason, they could present you with an accusation such as "Your profession directly causes low self-esteem in teenagers," and sit back to wait for your response. Cosmetic surgery can be a subject of both fascination and/or loathing, and depending on where the media is coming from in this instance they could go straight for the jugular. The question "Are you pressuring vulnerable women into spending money they don't have on procedures they don't need!?" has taken many forms over the years. We will talk about responding to difficult questions in the next section.

Editing

Of course there will always, ultimately, be a measure of editing involved—either on the radio, TV or print, this is part and parcel of producing a story. However, it is not that common to purposely and blatantly change the entire spirit of a quote by cutting it down. Naturally there will be always some editing but it won't be of the calibre of editing involved in, say, movie reviews! Where, for example, a magazine may say 'as exciting as watching paint dry' and the film poster will just quote them as having called it 'EXCITING ...'

It is worth noting, however, that there is recourse and if you feel that your words have been completely taken out of context, there are complaint bodies and these organizations can cost a journalist their career so they do take it seriously.

Mostly, however, journalists don't actually intend to twist your words BUT as I continue to reiterate, they *are* trying to produce a good story—one that will make their bosses happy, sell lots of papers and secure their job. Look, we're all human. So make it easy for them to begin with, and give them some good sound bites (more on that later).

PREPARING FOR THE INTERVIEW

Research the outlet

If it's with a magazine, pick up a copy at the news stand on your way home. Or have a flick through some back issues—perhaps your daughter or her friends will have a copy if it's a teenage girls' title. Is it a satirical magazine? Is it an august publication with an overt political leaning? What kind of writing or shows do they produce? Will they be taking a hard line or a light-hearted view?

Research the journalist

We covered some of this in the 'Pitching' section—Google is a magnificent tool for these opportunities. Drop into the conversation that you enjoyed their last article on the benefits of probiotics. Not being aware of the sort of thing they write has cost me dearly. I will never forget pitching a story to a national newspaper early in my career, and being so pleased they proved receptive that I didn't bother thoroughly researching the specific column that the reporter wrote every week. It was basically a sarcastic column poking fun at developments in the financial sector. My client was lightly lampooned, and while some would say that 'any publicity is better than no publicity' I was mortified and learnt my lesson. Whether it's *Marie Claire* or the *New York Times*, make sure also that it's a column or section that suits your premise. If it's a reactive PR opportunity, this is doubly important so you know what to expect and are 'forearmed'.

Research the audience

All media outlets know exactly who their audience is. It could be older women or teenage boys. They know exactly how much their viewers and readers earn. Find out—or get your publicist to find out—who their target audience is and whether it's appropriate for you. I once set up a breast surgeon to discuss the ideal breast proportions with the Playboy satellite radio station. An interview that was meant to be a 10-minute affair turned into a fantastically entertaining hour-and-a-half-long romp with Playboy Bunnies phoning in and submitting photos for evaluation. It wasn't an opportunity for everyone, but that particular surgeon rolled with it, and it couldn't have been a more perfect setting.

Think about the questions as well as the answers

> "Before I refuse to take your questions, I have an opening statement to make."
>
> —Ronald Reagan

It's worth repeating: put yourself in the interviewer's shoes. What would they want to know? Spend some time thinking about this before the interview—prepare any statements beforehand and don't be scared of putting them across first, then repeating them again at the end. It's very easy to get sidetracked with their questions but if you want to make a point, don't be afraid to make it and do it often. Most importantly—prepare sound bites ...

Preparing a sound bite

A sound bite should sum up your main point (whatever that may be) in simple, easy to hear terms that 'stick' in the ear, all in less than 20 seconds, and ideally in one sentence. Journalists will always be on the lookout for these, because they enhance their story and make it stand out. Editors and producers just don't have all day to spend talking to you, as entertaining as you are. Make sure they take little 'gems' away that will celebrate your awe-inspiring intellect and exalted wit.

First, decide what it is you want to say that will best illustrate your message (which hopefully you will have determined by now). Now we have to find a concise way of putting it across, which is best done via sound bites. Some useful tools to consider when crafting these are as follows:

- Alliteration
- Repetition
- Lists

If you're worried about being edited, use lists in your favour. Say something along the lines of "There are five things we must remember: A, B, C, D and E." It makes it very difficult for them to edit out because it would be weird to hear a radio interview where the expert says "A, C and E," or "1 and 4".

- Rule of 3

There is something magical about the number three—psychologically, it seems to 'stick' in the mind more. You can use this for repetition and lists.

- Word Play

If it comes naturally to you, then engage in word play. Journalists are mostly English majors!

- Humour

Again, feel free to engage in humour—it disarms people. If the situation is appropriate (and this is, needless to say, essential), make a joke. It will show that you don't take yourself too seriously.

- Current References

Quote a TV programme or a famous novel, whether it be *50 Shades of Grey or The Simpsons*.

- 'Borrow' from someone else

Take a famous quote and turn it on its head ("Ask not what your surgeon can do for you …")

- Think advertising slogan

DEALING WITH DIFFICULT QUESTIONS

When I speak at conferences or run workshops, this is usually the area I'm most asked about. The reality is some people deal fine with these situations, whereas others may struggle when facing hostility. I have worked with people that sail through straightforward interviews and come across as warm and engaging but as soon as they feel they're being attacked, they become flustered and stumble on their words. Journalists can sense this—it's like smelling fear. To be fair, they're not looking to humiliate anyone, they just want clear answers.

Funnily enough, the best people to learn from are, in fact, politicians. I don't mean of course subscribe to their particular morals or specific party leanings! But it's always interesting to watch how *they* deal with difficult questions, especially in debate situations. You will notice them using humour, you will see them making use of lists and rules of 3. Watch and learn from those Masters …

> *Tip: These tools also work for other public-speaking opportunities such as lecturing or speaking at conferences.*

Reflecting

Journalists hate this. They may come at you with an accusation or a statement that you know isn't true or accurate. You bounce the ball straight back in their court. They say to you: "We hear that X, Y or Z …"—you say: "Really, where have you heard this?" Or, they say "We've seen a study that says A, B and C," you say: "I'd be interested in seeing this report." Throw the ball back in their court.

Deflecting

This is a technique where you simply steer the answer to their question into more secure territory. For example, they might say something along the lines of "We believe that the public are concerned with X." You can bridge that by saying "Actually, what I have found in my practice is that patients are really wanting to know more about Y …" and expand.

No Comment

It is very rare that a good publicist will ever advise you to say 'no comment'. Put simply, it makes you look guilty or like you're trying to hide something. In some instances it's unavoidable, if specific legal cases can't be alluded to and so on, but most interviews you do will not be about those types of subjects. Whenever possible, try to structure a statement ahead of time and stick to it.

When Tragedy Strikes: The 3 Ps
You will see this trick of the trade being used often, especially when tragic events are covered in the news: Pity, Praise and Promise. You will note a politician or figurehead showing (1) sympathy: "Our thoughts and prayers are with the families," followed by (2) praise: "We would like to praise the efforts of the services involved who have worked tirelessly ..." concluded with (3) a promise to make things better: "We will be reviewing all procedures to ensure nothing like this ever happens again ..."

Over-talking

Counter-intuitively, there's not a lot to say about this—just keep going. Don't give them a chance to interrupt so just wax lyrical until they lose the will to live.

Practice

Practice, practice, practice (see what I did there? Rule of 3, Repetition ... Boom). The more you do interviews, the better you will be. Start with smaller ones if you're nervous, until you hit your groove. Like anything, you will become better with time.

Listen to others

Watch difficult interviews. Watch politicians and company CEOs and learn from the techniques they use.

The reality is that, if you really have to answer difficult questions, you can only use avoidance tactics for so long (to buy you some time). Eventually, however, you're better off addressing them head-on.

Here are some tips to keep in mind, depending on the type of interview you will be fielding.

What not to wear: these days, a lot of news programmes and chat shows find it boring to have people in business suits, and try to make the segments more dynamic by showing the experts 'in action' and in their own environment, such as their consulting rooms or even an operating theatre in hospital. It's more likely these days that if a clinician, they'll want you in scrubs or a white coat. There are, however, some rules that you should keep in mind if you find yourself being filmed. For example, you should always try to avoid very thin stripes on your shirt or dress, because they will 'strobe'. If the interview is in studio, find out about the screen behind you—when you see the Empire State building or Big Ben behind the newsreaders this is almost always a screen, which used to be mainly blue but nowadays they use green. So what will happen if it's a green screen and you *wear* green? You will appear as a disembodied head, perhaps with a City bus occasionally traversing your invisible torso. I've had to ask clients in the past to run out and get a new shirt or tie before heading into an impromptu interview.

Posture

Do as your mum always said, and don't slouch! Don't look too comfortable—especially when the interview takes place on a sofa, it will make you look like you're not being serious enough. On the other hand, there is no need to tensely perch on the edge of the seat, either. You'll just make the viewers anxious.

Animation/Semaphore

It is of course important to appear lively and warm, and not to come across as a robot. But also watch the hand movements don't get too animated, or it will look like you're engaging in semaphore signals. Also watch you don't find yourself fiddling with your watch or jewellery (speaking of which, tone down the flashy jewellery and brand logos). We all do things that we're unconscious of and the best option if you find yourself doing a lot of TV interviews is to play them back and observe—or if you're preparing for them, have someone film you. Better yet, undergo formal media training. The sessions my team runs always have TV segments where we record and critique back as a group what the interviewee is doing well and what they aren't.

Looking into the camera

It is extremely unusual to be asked to speak directly into the camera. Most of the time you will be facing an interviewer, but there are various scenarios in which this could take place. It may be in a TV studio with a presenter or newsreader present in the same room as you, or it could be done remotely from a regional or 'satellite' studio. In the latter case, you may be bundled into something vaguely resembling a broom closet, facing into a camera, which will project you onto a screen in another studio, where the presenters are based.

If the story allows, most TV crews (especially for news bulletins) will prefer to come to you, because it makes the segment much more visual if there is exciting equipment and shiny things around, making bleepy noises. In this type of situation there may be a presenter you will be addressing who will be off-camera, OR if they're short-handed the cameraman could even be the one asking the questions. If that is the case, they may ask you to address an imaginary spot to the side of the camera (the cameraman may wriggle a hand where you're supposed to be looking). In the U.K. they call this 'talking to Sooty [a hand puppet]', and it can be somewhat disconcerting. Feel free to discuss with them beforehand—it behoves them to get the best out of you.

Live/Pre-recorded

Always ask which one it is! There have been countless gaffes by people in the public eye who say something indiscreet because they do not realize they're still on air, or say live on the news "can we start again?" or accidentally catch themselves swearing. Always ask which it's going to be: if the interview is live, bottom line is you don't get a second chance and there's not much you can do about that—but if it's being pre-recorded, you can have more than one take. Having said that, they're not there for your benefit and they may not be keen to keep trying over and over until you're happy with what you're saying or how you sound. In the rare case you really want to start again and they seem resistant, pretend to cough or choke—but there's no need to throw yourself on the ground pretending to have a seizure or anything (just saying).

On location

Not only will they sometimes prefer to come to your premises, but occasionally you may find yourself having to do interviews out in the street or at a conference or trade show. In this instance, all the rules apply, but you will also have the added distraction of noise, passersby and probably colleagues who may be doing rude gestures behind the cameraman to get you to laugh. I am not making this up. You know who you are.

RADIO INTERVIEWS

Phone

The great majority of radio interviewers will *prefer* you to be in studio or via ISDN (digital transmission) line to truly guarantee sound quality and minimise the risk of interference or noise, but this isn't always possible. A lot of the time you will find yourself doing radio interviews from your phone, ideally from a landline rather than a cell phone. If the programme is live (see previous section), sometimes they can take place very early in the morning or late at night, depending on when they broadcast. I generally suggest to clients that regardless of the time or environment surrounding them, they smile while they're speaking (even if it feels a bit daft in an empty room), it really does make a difference in how you sound, and also stand up: this will make you sound more animated than if you're slumped in your favourite comfy chair.

In Studio/Down the line/Radio cars

Similarly to TV, you will ideally find yourself in the same room as the presenters, so you can address them directly. Occasionally they will come to interview you on location. Radio tries to be 'visual' as well, and seek background 'ambiance' noises as much as the next camera crew. I've even had a radio programme broadcast the sounds of liposuction taking place! Interviews in person can be—depending on the theme being discussed—fairly painless and potentially enjoyable, because there is a lot more interaction and you can respond to interviewer's body language signals. Occasionally though, you may find yourself 'down the line', which is basically another broom closet, this time with a microphone. They will give you headphones and you can answer questions from other studios or other locations. Sometimes there will be several interviews, one after the other, and they may even be asking the same questions if they're airing to a number of regional radio stations (this happens quite often with the BBC). Another option is a radio car, where you're sitting in a van and the interview is beamed via satellite. Depending on what's happening outside this can be a taxing situation, because a lot of people on the street will be fully aware that it is a radio or camera crew broadcasting from inside and could be extra noisy or even bang on the side of the vehicle, just for kicks. There's not a lot you can do about this unfortunately, just try and concentrate on the interview.

Phone-ins

Personally, I tend to caution clients against participating in phone-ins. Or, at least, I'm very careful about who I choose to face these, because we're dealing with a huge unknown. A phone-in segment generally entails taking calls and answering queries or comments from members of the public. Unlike researching an outlet or journalist, it's hard to predict what shape these enquiries might take. They could come from bored people, those with a bone to (publicly) pick, even disgruntled patients. There are only a handful of experts I consider so media-savvy that I would expose to this type of situation, not necessarily because they couldn't handle it but because publicists just aren't in the business of offering their own clients to be used as scapegoats. People out there can be a tiny bit … unpredictable, that's all. If you find yourself in the situation, try and address people's concerns directly (there's nowhere to hide), and if faced with difficult questions make free use of the techniques we covered in the previous section (reflect, deflect, over-talk …).

Giving good radio

If you 'give good radio', that is you're personable and use pithy sound bites that don't sound like you're talking down at people, the producers will want to have you time and again. It is a wildly underused medium, and a lot of people listen to the radio as part of their daily lives so it's certainly not to be sniffed at. Your local station may have some great opportunities to have a monthly programme, or to be a 'resident expert' (more on this later).

Know your audience

I cannot stress this enough. If the programme is aimed at 18–24 year olds, it's unlikely they will want to focus on facelifts. If it's a consumer affairs programme, they will have specific areas they will want to focus on, such as financing or advertising. Find out, and tailor your sound bites and answers accordingly, ahead of time. There is no point in giving a fantastic interview about baby boomer surgery to an audience of teenagers. And please, repeat with me: *you are not gangsta.* Don't even attempt to get down with da kidz. You have been warned.

PRINT INTERVIEWS

The main thing to keep in mind is that, yes, interviews taking place with a view to a print article may be slightly less pressurised and can usually be done from the comfort of your home, office or cell phone (only on some occasions do they bother with face-to-face). But just because they're in print it doesn't mean that the journalist will give you their copy ahead of time to review and approve. As mentioned in chapter 5, sometimes interviewees feel they have a right to vet what's been written, but the journalist (quite reasonably) feels they know how to do their job and they don't tell *you* how to do yours. Some journalists, however, might not mind running your quotes past you. It doesn't hurt to ask, but don't be offended if they refuse. They take their jobs as seriously as you take yours, so give them some credit.

Newspapers

The main thing to keep in mind about newspapers is how quick their turnarounds can be. They have to report on hundreds of news items everyday (or every week), and don't usually have time to do any of them in extreme depth. Understanding their constraints can be daunting, what they need they need now, and if you can't get back to them quickly they will simply move on to the next expert on their list. This is why it's so important acquire the ability to be able to throw together sound bites and offer views accurately and succinctly—help them sell papers, they will continue to use you for quotes.

Consumer and trade magazines

Fortunately magazines will have longer lead times than daily and Sunday newspapers, and will thus enjoy more time to thoroughly research a subject and be able to expand on it in more detail. Realising who they are writing for is, as always, invaluable. Monthly magazines have a 3–4-month lead time usually, which means that at the tail end of summer, they will be writing their bumper 'New Year, New You' issues. Keep in mind that if you make it into *Cosmopolitan* or *Men's Health* tomorrow, you will probably not see your name in lights for several months. Also, realise that May is too late for your 'Get your body bikini-ready' press release, because in all likelihood they will be working on September issues. Similarly, in August, they will be working on Festive Season and New Year editions and themes. This is of course monthlies—but weekly magazines, will also usually have a 3–4 week leads as well. The advantage with magazines is that they have less time pressures than with daily publications and the journalist will have more leeway to go back and forth with ideas with you, and explore additional angles.

The same time constraints with consumer magazines apply to trade publications, but keep in mind for interviews that trade publications *know their stuff*. These will be journalists who only write about cosmetic surgery, dermatology or aesthetic treatments. Trade outlets are much more difficult than consumer outlets in terms of interviews, because they will know what technical questions to ask. So prepare.

Deadlines

All journalists will have their own deadlines for a particular story and you—or your publicist—should always keep them in mind. Ignore at your peril! Sometimes, even if it's a daily newspaper, they will have a few days to get all their interviews in if it's an in-depth article. Many times I've asked clients to get back to me with an urgent answer when the deadline is the end of that day, and I receive a politely typed letter in the post from their secretary 2 weeks later, saying when they might be available to be interviewed at such and such time. A completely lost opportunity. Always ask when they need the answers/material by.

Images

If you have read the 'Press Kit' section, you will know that you should always have a number of materials at the ready and these include photos. There is no point in selling a fantastic new story about a new non-surgical treatment if you have no good quality, high-resolution before-and-after photos at hand. You should also always have a good photo of you, perhaps a couple of options: lecturing, even operating; photos of you in business wear, and/or in scrubs, because a lot of times the outlet that is quoting you will want your picture next to the piece. In some instances, the article may not even quote you directly but if it mentions a certain treatment and you have a relevant photo they can use, they will credit your clinic. It's a perfect chance to get a mention with very little work involved!

MEDIA INTERVIEW GUIDELINES

Before the interview

- Know the reporter, publication/programme, interview format, audience (ask your PR representative for a comprehensive brief)
- Know your goal for the interview, how you want your organisation to be portrayed. Draft any key messages you want to ensure come across
- Jot down likely questions, appropriate answers: hard and easy

During the interview

- Put your point across successfully: say it loud, say it clearly, say it first. Feel free to repeat at the end. Speak in 'headlines'
- Don't over-answer. Keep it short and snappy: use sound bites

- Less is more—know what not to say. Don't repeat inaccurate statements or accusations, especially when being filmed or recorded, because if that clip is shown (or it's the only bit a viewer catches), it sounds like you're agreeing with something that is negative
- Don't be fixated by the question. If necessary, 'deflect' to a related point
- Speak clearly. Avoid jargons and too-technical terms
- Don't get drawn in to saying more than you want to. Some journalists have a disconcerting gift of staring at you expectantly even though you've put your point across, and you might feel the pressure to keep going. This brings me to the next point:
- Know when to shut up or bring the interview to an end. Stop talking once you've said what you have to say. Feel free to bring the chat to a close in a friendly manner, by thanking them, getting up/shaking their hand
- Don't know the answer? Don't fake it. If appropriate, assure the reporter you will find and provide the needed facts in a timely manner, or offer to assist the reporter in finding the source (personally, I don't like to say 'no' to a journalist, I always say something along the lines of "I will get back to you on this.")
- Don't overlap the interviewer's question; begin your answer when the reporter is finished
- Don't speak 'off the record'—you are never off the record. Only some veteran publicists who are able to negotiate stories can afford to do this. Do not attempt.
- Keep cool. Don't be provoked!
- Run a mock interview beforehand if necessary
- Never lie to a reporter

11   Social media

Research from 2011 shows that nine out of ten doctors in the U.S. use social media for personal purposes. Online physician communities came up as the most popular sites, followed by LinkedIn, with Facebook and Twitter trailing behind.

http://www.ama-assn.org/amednews/2011/09/26/bil20926.htm

There are a number of guides and how-to manuals out there nowadays about Twitter, Facebook, LinkedIn, etc. so I will not endeavour here to teach you how to use them from a technical standpoint, but it would be absurd to ignore these possible and very direct channels of communication with the media. They can function as tremendous PR tools and enhance your credibility and make you—your practice, clinic or hospital—seem connected, interactive and responsive.

There are guidelines about doctors and social media regarding the separation of their personal and professional lives and I entreat you to follow those official, common-sense recommendations. There are published policies by the American and British Medical Associations (AMA and BMA), but the general gist is:

- Maintain patient confidentiality at all costs.
- Monitor your own Internet presence and be aware of your online image.
- If there is contact with patients, maintain appropriate boundaries.
- Keep personal and professional profiles separate.
- Defamation laws apply in either case.

AMA: http://www.ama-assn.org/ama/pub/meeting/professionalism-social-media.shtml

BMA: http://bma.org.uk/-/media/Files/PDFs/Practical%20advice%20at%20work/Ethics/socialmediaguidance.pdf

Recommendations I would make to anyone using social media apply to clinicians equally: treat Facebook personal pages like a family album, and accept only friends and family you know. To interact with patients, past and potential, on this platform (whilst maintaining ethical boundaries) build a 'business page' instead, which will enable you to interact with members of the public or media who choose to 'like' your company or clinic. From a marketing perspective, it does allow you to post news, and interact with people. It can create a sense of community, although rarely will it ever secure you more in the way of press coverage. It simply offers another channel of communication for a journalist to contact you should they wish to, or if they'd like to see what people say about you—however, it does take regular monitoring, as there is nothing sadder than an empty Facebook page. And be aware that such openness also means that people can leave negative reviews! So be cautious and react quickly by addressing any concerns directly.

Twitter, Facebook's younger, 'cooler' and rather more anarchic sibling, should be cautiously treated like an ongoing, water cooler-side conversation which you can dip in and dip out of. It does allow you to connect with people from areas you find of interest: from celebrities and sports figures to industry peers and relevant organisations. Over the last two years I have found more and more journalists who expect a 'Tweet' (basically a statement of no more than 140 characters) instead of a press release! Talk about having to be concise …

LinkedIn is probably the 'safest' option for you, if you fear the instant interaction that social media can demand. LinkedIn allows you to form groups with common interests, so you can still engage in conversations with like-minded individuals on a slightly more controlled platform. Treat your profile on LinkedIn like an online résumé/CV, and 'connect' with people you know or are aware of professionally. This builds up a network of connections with peers and companies of relevance, and can facilitate the formation of interesting groups and discussions.

The Web as a whole terrifies many doctors and it's not to be wondered at. But it's worth repeating the immortal Marketing adage: if you do not seek to position yourself, the public and your competitors will do it for you. Whether you choose to participate in social media or not, you probably have a presence there already or are being talked about (even if you're not aware of it). There are literally thousands of review sites and forums where—whether you like it or not—you, your clinic or services will be discussed. Just because you're not on Twitter and Facebook, doesn't mean you're not on Twitter and Facebook, if you get my drift. Use them and LinkedIn, if and as appropriate with your brand image.

> *Every point of contact reflects on your brand—whether it's your LinkedIn profile, your website or even the front door of your premises. Ensure all elements are in line with the image you wish to project.*

I'm not going to lie here—social media can be, on occasion, one big, nasty school playground where bullies abound. But to stress the point about media as a whole, you cannot ignore its existence and power. Over the last several years I've had to confront online detractors a handful of times and even consult lawyers more than once. One particular vicious journalist presented a tricky challenge by refusing to take calls or emails, and would only accept answers to accusatory questions in full public view on social media. If you manage these feeds efficiently, negative experiences should be extremely rare. A courteous response and an offer of help via phone or email make you look good, and detractors are the ones that could appear rude or uncompromising.

> *Internet trolls: People who post inflammatory, inappropriate or even outright insulting or devious comments on web pages, forums and discussions. Their only objective is to cause disruption.*

DISGRUNTLED PATIENTS

On more than one occasion I have found myself on client social media pages over a weekend or late night, immediately tackling any complaints that have appeared by offering a solution, help, or even just a friendly ear. I would rather feel they acknowledged and listened to than ignored, especially in full view of others.

> *Tip: Bad reviews or feedback are better addressed head-on. Ignoring them won't make them go away but actually fester, as they spread negativity.*

So why engage at all, when it can cause such aggravation, you may wonder? Negative comments would have made an appearance anyways, and I'm pleased for my clients that we are always online and able to address any issues immediately.

SOCIAL MEDIA CHECKLIST

- Make it part of your routine: one of the main complaints of doctors who don't want to engage in social media is 'they don't have the time'. Incorporate it in your daily schedule—for example, I check the pages first thing in the morning, just as I check the news headlines.
- Make liberal use of the mobile apps: Facebook, Twitter and LinkedIn are all available on your smartphone, that way you can have a quick skim in-between patients or while waiting for the OR.
- The key word here is engagement—constantly posting special offers and discounts without conversing with people will simply make you look like a spammer.
- Personalise and brand each of your sites: use your logo or even better a photo of yourself, don't just leave the anonymous Twitter 'egg'!
- Monitor your sites: Empty pages and feeds are magnets for spammers who will post their own competitions or inappropriate messages.
- Respond to people—if someone comes to you with a question or an observation, interact with them. Otherwise they'll think your practice or clinic may be equally unresponsive. If the comment is negative, thank them for their feedback and offer to tackle the issue.

- Don't criticise peers: this should be obvious! There's no such thing as 'deleting' something entirely from the Internet.
- Don't re-tweet or re-publish others' negative statements. By posting them, you're as responsible for what is being said as the person saying it.
- Don't get overwhelmed: there are free (yes, free!) tools that will help you manage your social media presence and post to LinkedIn, Facebook and Twitter, such as HootSuite and TweetDeck. Schedule yourself a half hour (it won't even take that long—you're a smart cookie) to choose and familiarise yourself with one.
- Have fun with it! The thing about social media is it's meant to be less formal. It's about conversations—how else could you find yourself chatting with a magazine editor in the U.K., a company CEO in Australia and a Hollywood movie star all over the course of a 10-minute lunch break or cab ride?

12 Conclusions

Is 'any publicity' REALLY 'good publicity'? Is every chance to speak to the media a positive opportunity? The only one who can answer what is ideal for your practice and brand is you. Review your objectives as an organisation or practitioner and determine what you really stand for. Your mission statement should dictate what kinds of press coverage you will seek and what kinds you will avoid. Are you comfortable discussing whether this or that celeb had this or that done? Do you want to participate in 'makeover' TV shows, or do you have a moral objection to them? With time, the media will learn what they can and can't get out of you. And let's not kid ourselves, there is always going to be a downside to exposure. The minute you say that black is black, someone else will pipe up and say that actually, *white* is black (remember Clarke's 4th law!). I won't say that everyone should engage in proactive PR activities if they don't wish to, but all cosmetic practitioners should at least have a modicum of understanding how it works—and indeed how it can do so in their favour.

> **CASE STUDY: The Boob Job Cream Saga**
>
> You may find that sticking your head above the parapet leaves you open to being attacked by others in the industry, in particular in a 'Wild West' environment that may contain little in the way of regulation. The minute you say "beware practitioners who do such-and-such," the practitioners who do such-and-such will be up in arms. In one memorable incident, a plastic surgeon was asked by a U.K. newspaper to comment on the claims made by a so-called boob job cream that promised the user increased

cup sizes when the product was rubbed in everyday. (I always wondered, wouldn't the hands get bigger as well?) The surgeon's view was that the public should exercise caution regarding these claims, as there was little scientific data backing them up. The response from the company was to issue a threat of a libel lawsuit. The Saga of the Boob Job Cream became a sort of 'cause celebre', with journalists leaping to the defence of the surgeon, free-speech organisations and even famous names such as Stephen Fry Tweeting their outrage. The matter was even debated in Parliament by MPs (somehow contributing to the words 'boob job cream' being bandied about in Westminster will remain for me a career milestone) when libel reform was discussed. The lawsuit was eventually dropped by the manufacturers, and as entertaining as such a public kerfuffle was, it was not pleasant for the surgeon who could have lost her livelihood through a lengthy and expensive legal trial.

There are downsides to speaking up. Your more snobbish colleagues may look down at you, and outspoken views may even land you in hot water (especially if you resemble Plain-Speaking Surgeon). Rivals may even seek to publicly attack you.

Many clinicians and professionals still wonder why we choose to engage with the media at all when it can be such a minefield, but the benefits can be far-reaching and above and beyond the enhancement of personal and business profiles. There is simply no other, more effective way, of reaching thousands if not millions of people and spreading the word on patient education and safety.

IS THIS THING WORKING?

As we have seen, there are many avenues to opening a dialogue with the media, and various ways of securing opportunities to engage with journalists and not all have to do with issuing press releases. In chapter 8 we discussed opportunities offered by speaking engagements such as conferences, seminars and consumer events as well as trade shows. Community engagement as well offers a strong face-to-face element that people will appreciate, because nothing can ever replace human interaction. Think of what's available to you: are there any opportunities to speak locally about skin cancer prevention, mole mapping, the latest advances in aesthetics? Offer to answer readers'/listeners' monthly questions in a woman's magazine or your local paper/radio station.

The more you are seen to interact with the press, the more they will seek you counsel and comments on developments in the sector. Eventually you may reach the exalted heights of every publicist's Holy Grail: the 'Resident Expert' role.

There are a variety of ways to monitor whether your PR efforts are proving successful or not. This will depend on the objectives you had before you launched the campaign: were you aiming to secure more business? Educate the public? Just raise your profile?

PR agencies will trot our buzz terms, such as ROI (return-on-investment) and AVE which basically stands for advertising equivalency. It boils down to what it would have cost you in advertising terms to secure the press interaction. However, it's a somewhat murky term, because it's hard to quantify the inherent trust that people place on media endorsement, which wouldn't be present in an ad or TV commercial. It is also difficult to establish a monetary value to the goodwill of journalists, who have come to rely on you for guidance.

One easy—and free—monitoring tool is Google Analytics, which will track the number of people visiting your website and how long they're 'sticking around' for. Use it liberally, and check how your stats are affected when you issued a press release or appear in a TV programme.

Oscar Wilde once said "The only thing worse than being talked about is not being talked about." I would posit that to establish whether PR working is pretty straightforward: as Mr. Wilde would be sure to concur, either you're being talked about, or you aren't!

*March 2010: The French manufacturing company Poly Implant Prosthèse (PIP) is placed in liquidation after the French medical safety agency recalls its breast implants.

*June 2010: Investigation reveals that industrial-grade silicone (apparently meant for mattresses) was being used in place of medical-grade silicone.

*September 2010: Tests show no cytotoxicity, but genotoxicity (effect on cell division) is 'inconclusive'.

*February 2011: It is discovered that the implants had also been sold under a different brand name around Europe.

*April 2011: Genotoxicity is ruled out.

*3 December 2011: A woman with PIP implants dies in France from a rare form of cancer, prompting a policy review and widespread press concern.

*23 December 2011: The French government recommends all French PIP implant patients seek their removal.

It was 9 pm on New Year's Eve 2011. I had one foot inside the bath, and the phone glued to my ear as I continued organising interviews on the unfolding PIP implants scandal. For the last few weeks, including weekends, Christmas and Boxing Day, I had been bombarding plastic surgeons with dozens of texts on a daily basis.

Can someone get to BBC Bristol by 4 pm?

Need a spokesperson for The Times.

Does anyone have any images of explanted PIPs?

Is anyone available for ITVs "This Morning"?

Despite what I suspect must have been growing resentment from spouses and families eager to enjoy festivities without a publicist's intrusive demands, surgeons from the British Association of Aesthetic Plastic Surgeons (BAAPS) rallied to cope with the demands of an increasingly fearful—if not outright hysterical—public and media.

I've been known to joke, when reviewing the list of spokespeople at our disposal, that we have unofficial categories such as 'think PR is beneath them' 'won't get out of bed for less than *Glamour'*, 'only science journals' and so on. And whilst it's true that to ensure our presence during this turbulent period I may have threatened some with bodily harm, and did not consider it beneath me to use tears, I only had to resort to these ignoble tactics once or twice: nearly all willingly stopped carving turkey and volunteered to help out. One surgeon who had never done a TV interview sat bravely on the BBC 'Breakfast' couch, another offered to drive halfway across the country through the night for a morning chat show when I couldn't find anyone local. No one pushed their own practice or website, or sulked because this person or that got more exposure—when it mattered, they stood up to be counted.

To truly comprehend how the BAAPS became the epicentre of information dispersal for all things PIP, we have to look back to when the rumblings of the scandal first started making their way from France in early 2010. With every development—from the company's liquidation to the revelation that the gel within the implants was meant for mattresses—we faced the dilemma: do we notify the media? There is not always consensus in being the first to break certain news. MANY times I'm asked by clients "Does everyone need to find out about this?" "Do we really need to be the ones bringing attention to it?" In this instance, there could only be one answer.

Anytime there is damaging information, publicists have to weigh up the options. Is it better to select a specific newspaper and trust they will write something sensible which will include our advice? Or wait until someone else gets ahold of the information (which they undoubtedly will) and we lose all control over what is being said?

And so, we issued press releases when the first tests were delayed because the samples had been impounded; when it was discovered the protective shell had been dispensed with; when the first genotoxicity tests were 'inconclusive' and, as early as February 2011, announced that cosmetic surgery tourists may unwittingly have received PIP implants under a different brand name. Journalists, and the public via social media, came to rely on the BAAPS to stay informed.

Once France announced they would remove all PIP implants, the media onslaught was relentless. At the time, the U.K. government's stance remained broadly along the lines of "nothing to see here, folks," but the women sobbing on the phone and writing panicked emails clearly felt otherwise. In the midst of a sea of rumours, confusion and slow reactions, the BAAPS directive was unequivocal and consistent throughout. There was no immediate danger but it was the surgeons' expert opinion that the implants should come out, and preferably before rupture. It was important to reassure and educate as many as possible.

In December 2011 and January 2012, the BAAPS appeared in over 1,500 articles and news bulletins from outlets such as the BBC, Al Jazeera, Daily Mail, Financial Times, Guardian, Telegraph to France 24, Wall Street Journal and the New York Times.

Although it is true that, after nearly a decade of working together—going onto the sixth Presidential term now—the BAAPS and its Press Office function like a well-oiled machine, there are a few basic principles that have ensured their message (whether it be PIPs, moobs or a proposal for regulations), nearly always goes stratospheric.

1. They understand that having a PR agency is like paying for a gym membership. Many organisations fail to understand that just by virtue of paying a retainer, publicists cannot 'magic' coverage out of thin air. They have to invest the time and effort—and be ready to receive many (probably annoying) texts and emails demanding immediate response.
2. As a publicist, I'm only as good as what I'm given. A succession of BAAPS Presidents and their Councils have understood the importance of clearly articulated messages, and never fail to provide a solid direction and 'party line'.
3. The decision to break a story is always a difficult one: in PR there are no guarantees. Even the journalist writing the story doesn't know—and has no input—on what the headline will ultimately be. If you want to control exactly what will be said and who will be quoted, book an advert.

If used well, the media can be a health care organisation's most valuable mouthpiece. In this instance the willingness of scores of surgeons provided a direct line of help and information to the victims of this ongoing scandal—because even the best PR machine cannot create something out of nothing. The saga continues …

*18 June 2012: The final PIP report shows no evidence of long-term health damage; the U.K. government reiterates its position that there is no need for routine explanation, but calls upon all providers to offer the option of removal if the patient wishes.

Index

Advertisements in public relations, 13
Advertising
  awareness and, 15
  in cosmetic surgery, 10
  versus editorial, 16–17
  versus public relations, 15
Advertising *versus* editorial public
    relations, 15, 16–17
Aesthetic professionals, 7
Aesthetic treatments, 1, 4, 7, 21
AIDA. *See* Awareness, Interest, Desire
    and Action
American Medical Associations (AMA),
    104–105
Awareness, advertising and, 15
Audience, knowing, 50–59, 91–92
  blogs, 58
  consumer health, 57
  creating media list, 59
  men and women's audience, 56–57
  national *versus* local press, 51–53
  other specialist magazines, 57–58
  overview, 50
  in radio interviews, 100
  trade *versus* consumer press, 53–54
Awareness, Interest, Desire and Action
    (AIDA)
  in marketing, 15

BAAPS. *See* British Association of
    Aesthetic Plastic Surgeons
Boilerplates, press releases, 68
Blackberry Botox, 3
Blogs, 58
BMA. *See* British Medical Associations
Botox, 54

Branding, real, 12
Breast cancer, awareness, 53
British Academy of Cosmetic
    Dentistry, 1
British Association of Aesthetic Plastic
    Surgeons (BAAPS), 1, 112–115
British Medical Associations (BMA),
    104–105

Case studies
  cosmetic surgery, 21–25
    ear implant, 21–22
    PR blunder, 22–23
    teen surgery, 24–25
  proactive PR
    'any publicity is good publicity'
        approach, 29
  on reactive PR, 21–25
    ear implant, 21–22
    PR blunder, 22–23
    teen surgery, 24–25
  media and, 109–110
  newsworthy, 39–49
    consent for, 43
    consumer *versus* professional/trade
        press, 43
    examples, 43–46
    free/discounted procedure for
        publicity, 46–47
    informed decision in, 41
    interviews and, 42–43
    journalists as, 47–48
    making good, 41
    other angles, 48–49
    payment of stories of, 42
    photography in, 42

Case studies (*Continued*)
   plastering photos of celebs and,
      48–49
   sourcing, 40
   things to be noted in, 41–42
   using employees as, 47
   versus testimonals, 40
Celebrity doctors, 9–11
Celebrity endorsement, 13
Checklist
   for case studies, 46
   for new procedure and
      techniques, 35
   for social media, 107–108
   for trends, 38
Clarke's 4th Law, 24
Collagen marshmallows, 20
Commissioning editors, 74, 75
Community engagement, 110
Consent for case studies, 43
Consumer health
   audience and, 57
Consumer press, trade *versus,* 53–55
Consumer *versus* professional/trade
      press, 43
Controlling copy, journalist and, 28
Cosmetic surgery, advertising and
      marketing in, 10
Cosmetic surgery publicist, 1–4
Cost differences in public relations, 13
Courting controversy, defined, 29

Difficult questions, interview, 93–95
   deflecting, 94
   no comment, 94–95
   others, listen to, 95
   over-talking, 95
   practice, 95
   reflecting, 94

Ear implantation, 21–22
Ear reconstruction, new technique in,
      33–35
Experts, note on other, 28–29

Facebook, 9, 22
Financial Times, 5
Foster relationships with writers and
      editors, 27

Gibson's Law, 24
Golden Triangle of health care, 27–28, 32
Google Analytics, 111

Hello!, 13
Human interest, 27

Interview, 85–88
  accusations, 90
  aggressive questions, 88–89
  difficult questions, dealing with,
     93–95
  editing, measure of, 90–91
  friendly questions, 88
  media interview guidelines, 102–103
  preparing for, 91–93
  print, 100–102
  radio, 98–100
  repeated questions, 89–90
  TV, 96–98

Journalist, 7
  as case studies, 47–48
  close relations with, 24
  controlling copy and, 28
  interviews by, 42–43
  researching, 91
  specialized areas of, 53–54
Journalists, pitching to, 73–84
  DIY PR, 81–82
  exclusives, 82–83
  newswires, 83–84
  press release distribution services,
     83–84
  search engine optimisation, 83–84
  staff *vs.* freelancers, 81

Knowing your audience. *See* Audience

Lip enhancement procedure, 34–35
Liposuction, 54
Local, national *versus,* 51–53

Magazines
  men and women's, 56–57
  other specialist, 57–58
Marie Claire, 13
Marketing mix strategies, 14–17
  online and offline, 14

Media coverage
  human interest, 27
  new procedures, techniques or
    technology, 27
  statistics and trends, 27
Media enquiries on cosmetic surgery,
    18–20
Media
  cost differences in, 13
  endorsement, 12
  needs, 8–9
  newsworthy and, 32
  plastering photos of celebs and,
    48–49
  proactive coverage and, 29–30
  and thinking of, 30
Media briefings, 68–72
Media, downside of, 109
Media interview guidelines, 102–103
  before the interview, 102
  during the interview, 102–103
Men's magazine, 56–57
Miami Thong Lift, 3

National *versus* local, 51–53
  case studies, 52–53
New procedures and techniques, 33–35
New York Times, 13
Newswires, 83–84
Newsworthy, 27, 31–49
  case studies, spot a, 39–49
  human interest, 39
  media and, 32
  new procedures and techniques,
    33–35
  studies, statistics and trends, 35–38

Opening paragraphs, press releases,
    65–66
Opportunities, reactive PR, 25–26
Otoplasty, 33

Payment for stories of case studies, 42
Personal selling, 15–16
Photography in publications, 4
PIP. *See* Poly Implant Prosthèse
Poly Implant Prosthèse (PIP) crisis, 18,
    112–115
PR. *See* Public relations

PR agency, reasons to hire, 8
Preparation, for interview, 91–93
  audience, research, 91–92
  journalist, research, 91
  outlet, research, 91
  questions and answers, 92
  sound bite, 92–93
Press release distribution services,
    83–84
Press releases, 62–68
  boilerplates, 68
  examples, 64
  opening paragraphs, 65–66
  quotes, 66–68
Print interviews, 100–102
  consumer and trade magazines,
    101
  deadlines, journalists, 101–102
  images, 102
  newspapers, 100–101
Proactive PR, 5, 27–30
  case study, 29
  controlling copy, 28
  'Golden Triangle' themes of health
    care, 27
  note on other experts, 28–29
Public relations (PR), 13. *See also*
    Specific topics
  advertisements in, 13
  aesthetic treatments and, 7
  celebrity doctors and, 9–11
  cost differences in, 13
  illustrations for, 12
  in health care, 13
  needs of, 8–9
  reasons for hiring agency, 8, 10–11
  rules and guidelines for, 12
  strategies of, 8
Public relations campaigns, 2
  media briefings, 68–72
  press kit, 60–61
  press releases, 62–68
  start-up materials, 61

Quotes, press releases, 66–68

Radio interviews, 98–100
  audience, knowing, 100
  'give good radio,' 99–100

Radio interviews (*Continued*)
  phone, 98
  phone-ins, 99
  in studio/down the line/radio cars,
    98–99
Reactive media relations, 5
Reactive PR, 18–26
  defined, 20
  involves, 18
  long-term relationships with, 25
  opportunities, 25–26
Re-plumping effect, 35
Revenge surgery, 3

Search engine optimisation (SEO),
    83–84
SEO. *See* Search engine optimisation
Social media, 104–108
  checklist, 107–108
  disgruntled patients, 107

Staff *vs.* freelancers, journalists, 81
Statistics and trends, 27

Teen surgery, 24–25
Testimonals, case studies versus, 40
Tooth decay, 5
Trade *versus* consumer press, 53–55
Trust on media, 13
TV interviews, 96–98
  animation/semaphore, 96–97
  camera, looking, 97
  Live/pre-recorded, 97–98
  location, 98
  posture, 96
Twitter, 9, 22

Using employees as case studies, 47

Wild West analogy, 10
Women's magazine, 56–57